"Babies Need Mothers"

Cover flaps from the

Inside front cover flap:

Sometimes what is most profound profoundly simple once revealed. This mig apply to concepts found in this book.

New understanding is presented with such simplicity that a child can comprehend, and it is changing the thinking of renown leaders in the field.

A simple process is hypothesized, one that everyone already knows, one for which twelve precise parallels are drawn, one that is backed with significant data.

Did the brightest minds, the costliest research, the mountains of peer-reviewed literature and the billions of research dollars fail to make the critical distinction between cause and effect?

Could this possibly be?

Evaluate this for yourself and see. If indeed a true cause has been identified, then true prevention is made possible, for the first time.

Schizophrenia, depression, ADHD, school violence, autism, symbiosis, drug and alcohol dependence, eating disorders, bipolar disorder, borderline personality disorder and more, might fall into the ranks of what can be prevented, and prevented at three levels: 1. prevention of origin, very early in life, 2. prevention of a first breakdown later in life, 3. prevention of a recurrence, based on new understanding of origin and mechanism.

videly
iding
...ms and treatment of schizophrenia. He graduated from the University of Michigan School of Medicine in 1962, and then focused his attention on the study of the human mind.

Dr. McKenzie acquired valuable knowledge about the complex realm of mental illness while studying at the Menninger School of Psychiatry, followed by several years of training at the Philadelphia Psychiatric Center and the Philadelphia Psychoanalytic Institute.

In 1986 Dr. McKenzie was nominated for the Dana Award for Pioneering Achievements in Health.

In 1996, Dr. McKenzie wrote a textbook – *Delayed Posttraumatic Stress Disorders From Infancy: The Two Trauma Mechanism* – with co-author Dr. Lance Wright.

Dr. McKenzie's deep commitment to serving people was recognized when he was awarded Temple University's Nelson and Winnie Mandela's Humanitarian Award for his outstanding devotion to patients suffering from the effects of schizophrenia.

Since 1966, Dr. McKenzie has studied the relationship between trauma and Schizophrenia. Through the years he has dedicated himself to the evaluation and analysis of trauma and its immediate and long-range effects on behavior and mental health.

"Babies Need Mothers"

How Mothers Can Prevent Mental Illness in their Children

Clancy D. McKenzie, M.D.

Copyright © 2009 by Clancy D. McKenzie, M.D.

Library of Congress Control Number: 2008904542
ISBN: Hardcover   978-1-4363-4308-4
               Softcover   978-1-4363-4307-7

All rights reserved. No part of this book may be reproduced or transmitted in any form or by any means, electronic or mechanical, including photocopying, recording, or by any information storage and retrieval system, without permission in writing from the copyright owner.

Library of Congress Cataloging-in-Publication Data

McKenzie, Clancy, 1936—

p. "Babies Need Mothers" How Mothers Can Prevent Mental Illness in their Children/ Clancy McKenzie.—1st ed. cm.

Includes index.

1. Mental Illness—Cause, prevention, treatment. 2. Schizophrenia. 3. Depression. 4. Bipolar disorder. 5. Addiction. 6. Alcohol, drug dependence. 7. School violence. 8. Borderline personality disorder. 9. Attention deficit hyperactive disorder (ADHD). 10. Autism, symbiosis. 12. Religion, God, spirituality. 13. Enlightenment. 14. Meditation. 15. Dreams, "programmed" dreams. 16. Visions. 17. Love. 18. Need, desire. 19. Babies. 20. Mothers. 21. Child-rearing.

1. Title

Published in the United States by Xlibris, a strategic partner of Random House Ventures, LLC, a subsidiary of Random House, Inc.

Printed and bound in the United States of America.
August 2009. Final editing June 21, 2010
First Edition

10 9 8 7 6 5 4 3 2 1

To order additional copies of this book, contact
Xlibris Corporation
1-888-795-4274
www.Xlibris.com
Orders@Xlibris.com
47117

For next day shipping and autographed copies, order through www.DrMcKenzie.com or BabiesNeedMothers.com

CONTENTS

Acknowledgements..vii
Preface..xvii
Chapter 1   Search For Cause..3
Chapter 2   Having Schizophrenia Is Unnecessary 11
Chapter 3   Diagrams of Schizophrenia and Delayed
             Posttraumatic Stress Disorder from Adult Life.................23
Chapter 4   Does Schizophrenia Meet the Diagnostic Criteria for
             Delayed Posttraumatic Stress Disorder?.............................44
Chapter 5   Background: Autobiographical Sketch........................57
Chapter 6   A Guided Journey?..61
Chapter 7   Amazing Spiritual Gifts of Others.....................78
Chapter 8   The Cornerstone that the Builders Rejected.................87
Chapter 9   Brief Review Plus Age of Origin of
             Other Early Parameters 95
Chapter 10   Other Searches for Cause 106
Chapter 11   Age of Origin of Other Symptoms and
             Diagnostic Categories 116
Chapter 12   Age of Origin of Other Delayed
             Posttraumatic Stress Disorders..........................126
Chapter 13   Prevention of Serious Mental and Emotional Disorders 143
Chapter 14   The Primary Treatment Principles for
             Patient and Therapist....................................148
Chapter 15   Psychotherapy with Psychotic Patients 176
Chapter 16   Other Treatment Modalities.............................183
Chapter 17   Meditation...195
Chapter 18   Love Energy: The Life Force and
             The Fountain of Youth..................................204
Chapter 19   Programmed Dreams 222
Chapter 20   Babies Need Mother's Love 253
Appendix..263
Index..289

Acknowledgements

Throughout my journey in the field of psychiatry, there have been many teachers, friends and colleagues who have contributed along the way. By far the most helpful was **Dr. O. Spurgeon English**, first as training analyst and then friend and neighbor. For thirty years we discussed all new findings and concepts and he reviewed everything I wrote, adding pearls of wisdom along the way. While others were quick to dismiss new ideas, he encouraged every one of them. Shortly before his passing, he smiled when I told him his Foreword to the textbook might usher psychiatry into the 21st Century. That thought was pleasing to him. His last words to me were "I wish I had discovered that."

Dr. Lance S. Wright was another special friend and teacher who was instrumental in the growth and development of the findings. He provided a background of sound psychodynamic theory and kept me abreast of developments in the field, as I busied myself searching for cause, treatment and prevention of mental illness. He conducted several original research studies. **Dr. Sarnoff Mednick** surveyed for me the 6,000 persons with schizophrenia in the Finnish database, and **Dr. Preben Bo Mortensen** provided me with data on 2,669 people in the Danish cohort on schizophrenia. I would not have been able to conduct such large studies myself. **Dr. Viktor Frankl** taught me to add new meaning to the patient's life, which I never have forgotten. **Dr. John Rosen** was helpful in adding his knowledge and approach to treating schizophrenia, and **Dr. Margaret Mahler** provided the first clue to the origin of childhood schizophrenia, which was instrumental for later discoveries. **Dr. John DeCani**, department chair of statistics at Wharton Business School, approved my original research design and statistical analysis of data that confirmed the origin of schizophrenia. **Dr. John Nash** also proved helpful in our many long discussions.

In recent years, several noted psychoanalysts have been most helpful. **Dr. Harold Stern** was in charge of a schizophrenia conference at Jefferson University when I called to see if there was room on the roster to speak. "It's been filled for three months" he replied. In the next few minutes I explained my findings. He immediately recognized the paradigm-changing significance and said "we'll *make* room for you on the schedule." We have been exchanging ideas ever since, and he really understands this process.

I also owe much to **Dr. Brian Koehler** who has a remarkable ability to crystallize the essence of the latest technological discoveries to the depths of psychoanalytic literature. I doubt that I have ever known a person with equal capabilities. **Prof. Wilfried Ver Eecke** is another expert with whom I have had lively discussions regarding the origin and mechanisms of mental illness. **Koehler** and **Ver Eecke** were both quick to recognize the merits of the work described in this book, and they use my textbook, written with **Dr. Lance Wright**, for teaching purposes in New York University and Georgetown University respectively. Another person from whom I learned a truly unique psychoanalytic approach for the treatment of schizophrenia is **Dr. Ira Steinman**. He is known for his remarkable ability to engage the psychotic patient through the patient's associations to delusional ideation. Two others have contributed their unique ways of engaging patients to bring them out of psychosis: **Dr. Jack Rosberg** and **Dr. Al Honig**. Both studied with John Rosen and carry forward some of his insights and techniques. Honig developed a cottage group or home away from home approach that fits in well with the treatment modalities I have pioneered. **Dr. Grace Jackson**, one of the brightest persons in the field, brings in-depth knowledge of the side effects of medications. She has been a valuable resource for patients who have been prescribed dangerous combinations of powerful mind-altering drugs. Another bright light in the field is **Dr. Bert Karon**, a pioneer of psychotherapy for schizophrenia.

It is not possible to include the name of every medical professional who has contributed to my efforts to bring prevention and treatment to those in need, but each of the ones mentioned above has one thing in common: each has great love and compassion for patient and family. It is this love that is the source of their enlightenment, and the power behind their efforts.

I am also indebted to those who have taught me meditation and spiritual practices that have enabled me to see what otherwise would have remained hidden. These teachers have been people of different races and faiths, from all continents and walks of life. In particular, I am deeply grateful to **Dr. Orest Bedrij**, who has provided his wisdom and phenomenal insight, as well as his unwavering support for nearly a quarter of a century.

To properly and fully acknowledge my incredible wife, **Dianna**, and our two precious daughters, **Victoria** and **Christina**, would require a volume without end. For two years, after spending long hours in the office each day, I devoted nearly all free time to the preparation of this book. My family's unwavering support, their faith and confidence in me, has been the fuel of my existence.

Lastly, I am grateful for the help of many who participated in editing and making suggestions for the manuscript, including **Dr. Bob Novak, Michael David Severson, Charles Bubar, Meg Switzgable, Peggy Deardorf**, and my primary editor, to whom I am especially indebted, **Ben Dati**. His suggestions were particularly helpful in making the book acceptable to widely divergent groups of individuals—from scientists to philosophers to spiritual leaders from all denominations and religions.

Endorsements

Dr. McKenzie's new book is a rare example of careful conceptual reasoning about basic categories in medicine. Ultimately this is what is sorely needed in rational thinking about the mysteries of mental illness. This book is a fascinating contribution and well worth reading, precisely because it upsets the applecart. I recommend it to anyone who wants to get beyond rigid categorization in psychiatry and look at enduring problems of the mind in new ways.

Raymond Moody
Author, Life After Life;
MD, PsyD, PhD philosophy

Psychiatry has become, in my opinion, too much of the idea of merely "drugs and observations," and of course this pattern can be considered in relation to the profits made by the companies developing and selling the drugs. I endorse broader considerations in psychiatry, such as Dr. McKenzie proposes.

John F. Nash, Jr.
Nobel Laureate

Dr. McKenzie's book is revolutionary. Some long sought answers to causes of psychosis and other severe mental illnesses are explained in clear and understandable language. He not only describes cause and effect, but also provides remedies for healing that are unique and long lasting. He shows clearly and unmistakably the way to recover health, and his findings could change the prevailing way of treating chronic mental difficulties.

Harold Stern, PhD, Psychoanalyst

Old theories of modern science literally melt away before the riveting and crystal clear logic that erases any thought of current hypotheses.

Dr. Stephen Levine, Scientist, Author

This book is rich in new ideas that are a further development of the enlightening, stimulative and provocative ideas described in his earlier book with Lance S. Wright, MD: *Delayed Posttraumatic Stress Disorders from Infancy: The Two Trauma Mechanism*. I have used this latter book in my courses at Georgetown University and I plan to continue to use the ideas of Dr. McKenzie in my classes. No one will regret reading this book.

Wilfried Ver Eecke, Professor in Philosophy
Adjunct Professor in Psychology
Georgetown University

It is more effective to teach people how to drive safely than to repair smashed cars. Likewise, it is more effective to teach parents how to prevent mental illness in their children than to repair their damaged lives. Modern psychiatry is concerned with the treatment of mental diseases and disorders. Now, in his breakthrough research, Dr. McKenzie has identified the origin of serious mental and emotional disorders, and has discovered how mothers, through a loving and caring approach, can actually prevent these illnesses from ever occurring. Just as Albert Einstein's contributions were a quantum leap beyond Newtonian physics, so Dr. McKenzie's contribution to understanding cause is a quantum leap beyond present theories. This allows for true prevention for the first time.

Dr. Orest Bedrij, Author of
'1': The Foundation and Mathematization of Physics

My research for a movie brought my attention to Dr. McKenzie. Like many persons ahead of their time, Dr. McKenzie is sometimes viewed as a threat to others in his field. This is unfortunate because clearly his means of prevention could eliminate a very large portion of mental illness in this country and worldwide. His work is readily understood by professionals and laypersons alike. He has received high endorsements from members of the US Senate and Congress. A number of top professionals, who thoroughly reviewed his work, consider his findings to represent one of the greatest breakthroughs in psychiatry in the second half of the 20th Century.

Meg Switzgable
Independent Director/Producer
Documentaries on 60 Minutes and PBS Frontline

What is schizophrenia? Is it one thing or a combination of important issues beginning at the earliest part of life? Dr. McKenzie pulls together in a brilliant manner the issues comprising schizophrenia and gives us a greater understanding of the condition. I have been treating this condition for 54 years, and Dr. McKenzie has offered me a better understanding of the issues. I think this book is a must for the profession. Rarely mentioned elsewhere, is the importance of caring (loving) by the psychotherapist. I thought this was the basic issue, and Dr. McKenzie makes a special point of it.

Jack Rosberg, PsyD
Director, Anne Sippi Clinic and Foundation

This book is a 'tour de force' in its originality, basic scientific and biological approach, and its potential for preventive treatment of psychosis.

Kurt N. Langston, MD, Psychiatrist

A Voice out of the Past

It is with pleasure that I write this endorsement of Dr. McKenzie and his many years of fruitful and creative work. I have known Dr. McKenzie initially as one of his instructors, 35 years ago, in his training, and then as a friend and a co-author of various publications. As a clinical teacher of Psychiatric Residents in child, adolescent and adult psychiatry at Hahneman Medical University and at the Department of Psychiatry at the University of Pennsylvania, I was very familiar with academic literature and research. As our collegial work expanded, I provided a productive critical balance for Dr. McKenzie's creative flair and I recognized that we had a uniquely productive relationship. As a Board Certified Psychoanalyst of Adults, Children and Adolescents I presented a sound psychodynamic framework which helped to structure new observations.

What Dr. McKenzie has uncovered is very unique to the field of psychiatry, and possibly represents one of the greatest breakthroughs, if not the greatest breakthrough, in the second half of the 20th Century.

He has identified unsuspected infant separation traumas in the first two years of life, which correlate with the later development of schizophrenia. This has been confirmed by independent research on data from 9,000 persons with schizophrenia. What this indicates is that Trauma in early developmental stages of a child can have on going psychodynamic and structural effects as development continues. This new view opens more accurate understanding of the complexity of cause and reveals more opportunities for effective intervention and promotion of healing and getting back on track of maturational development.

As a result of this pioneering work, primary prevention of most serious disorders is possible for the first time.

He has expanded the concepts to include a wide range of infant traumas, and a wide range of disease entities that are specific to the particular age traumatized. He further has identified the precipitating mechanism for the initial onset of the disorder, which allows for a second level of prevention—i.e., prevention of an initial psychosis or major depression in the vulnerable teenager or young adult.

Additionally, based on our new understanding of origin and mechanisms derived from the clinical observations and research study, effective new treatment methods are possible. This is the third level of prevention—i.e., prevention of a recurrence among those who already have the disorder.

For many years he submitted nothing for peer review because he had no peers to review this totally new work. Only persons at the highest levels—who were beyond conducting peer reviews—were able to recognize the magnitude of the work. As such, various leaders in the field, including Anna Freud, Erik Erickson, Bruno Bettelheim, Hanns Strupp of Vanderbilt, Peter Sifneos of Harvard, O. Spurgeon English of Temple and other notables wrote letters of high praise and endorsement. For example, in 1984 Dr. Paul MacLean, Chief of Brain Evolution and Behavior at NIMH, wrote that he concurred with where and how the schizophrenic process was taking place in the brain, and he stated that the work went beyond the Child Development theories of Margaret Mahler. Thus a leading brain researcher agreed with not only the biological aspects of the theory, but stated the work went beyond that of the leading psychological theorist as well.

In 1993, O. Spurgeon English, Department Chairman at Temple University for 34 years, wrote: "The concepts presented are based on sound psychodynamic principles supported by findings in the literature. Theory is a marriage between psychological and biological, spanning the neuroses and the psychoses, from infancy to old age. It identifies mental illness as one mechanism, and psychology and biology as one process. As such, it is the beginning of a new unification theory of mental illness."

Thus it is clear, from the endorsements of the top scholars of our times, and from my personal review and interaction with him on all levels of the work, that this pioneering work is of highest creativity and highest quality, and that it offers much to mankind in that for the first time there can be primary prevention of serious mental and emotional disorders.

Lance S. Wright, MD
October 10, 2000

Reviews from cover of Textbook:

DELAYED POSTTRAUMATIC STRESS DISORDERS FROM INFANCY

The Two Trauma Mechanism
_____

Clancy D. McKenzie, MD
and
Lance S. Wright, MD

This book breaks with traditional thinking from the first paragraph . . . offers an alternative to viewing, treating, managing and preventing serious emotional disorders . . . breaks ground in suggesting the role of early trauma in accounting for mental disorders throughout the life cycle, in identifying the *two trauma mechanism,* and in the conceptualization of early traumatic events relating to the development of Borderlines, Schizophrenia, PTSD, Autism, Symbiosis and other disorders—forcing academics to reevaluate our thinking. The research is respectable, adds to their arguments and is in support of their model.

—**Charles F. Figley**, Psychosocial Stress Research Program, Florida State University

I was very skeptical about [Dr. McKenzie's] findings, but the Finnish database on 6,000 schizophrenic patients revealed a very high level of statistical significance. We confirmed a substantially higher rate of schizophrenia among those with siblings less than two years younger.

—**Sarnoff Mednick**, Social Science Research Institute University of Southern California

The concepts presented are based on sound psychodynamic principles supported by findings in the literature. Theory is a marriage between psychological and biological, spanning the neuroses and psychoses, from infancy to old age. It identifies mental illness as one mechanism, and psychology and biology as one process. As such, it is the beginning of a new unification theory of mental illness.

—**O. Spurgeon English**, formerly of Temple University

Through literature review and their own research, Drs. McKenzie and Wright demonstrate the profound relationship between early infant trauma and the later development of serious emotional disorders. Evidence of early traumatic origin may soon be recognized as one of the most important research findings in recent decades. This model goes beyond prevalent thinking to show that biological research only measures the results of the disease process and does not address the origins of mental illness. This book identifies primary prevention and offers new treatment methods based on the recognition of the *two trauma mechanism.*

—**Gordon and Breach**

Preface

You will read of many new concepts throughout this book, but they did not come through deductive reasoning alone, and it would be wrong to portray them that way. Many came through flashes of insight, coincidences, synchronicities, visions during the night, dreams, "programmed" dreams, meditation and words spoken during sleep. Only later were these glimpses of truth confirmed by logic, careful analysis and mathematical calculation.

This is not something foreign to science, but rarely is it acknowledged. Albert Einstein intuitively knew $E = MC^2$ twenty years before he was able to prove it. German scientist Friedrich August Kekulé first saw the benzene ring in a daydream, and Sigmund Freud wrote that if he logically thought one thing but intuitively sensed another, he followed his intuition.

It is important to reveal how the information was received. To the young scientist this could be more important than the information itself. The fuel for discovery was total compassion for patient and family, with no other motive whatsoever.

Learning to tap into knowledge that already is fully present in the universe need not be a formidable task. For this reason we include an autobiographical sketch to provide personal background, and then describe events leading to the process of discovery, encounters with others who relied on information gathered beyond the five senses, and then strong resistance encountered to revelation material.

The risk is that if some of the accounts are beyond the range of experience of the reader, he or she might dismiss the more important aspects of this work. For others they will have great meaning, and without them no amount of scientific investigation would hold validity.

It is important that everyone understands the scientific findings, with full appreciation of their significance. These findings make it possible to eliminate many serious mental and emotional disorders, and thereby reduce the suffering of countless families worldwide. We would not want any reader to dismiss the actual data and relevant conclusions because of strong convictions one way or another. Nowhere is the reader told what to believe. All experiences are simply reported as data. Science is open exploration. In the interest of science, let us explore this data together.

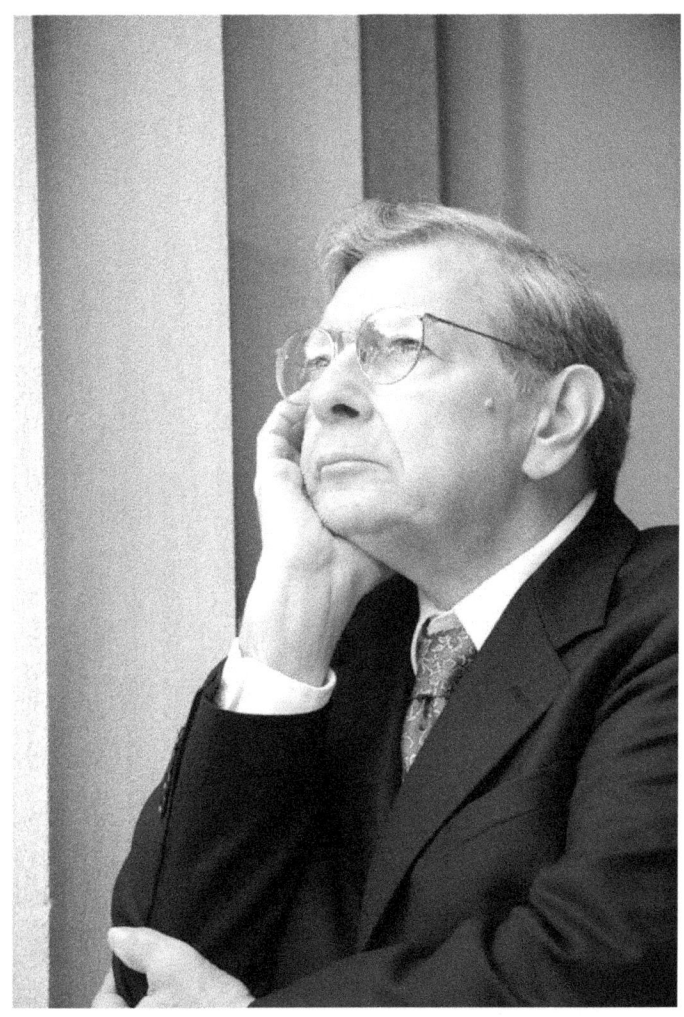

Author, at Philadelphia's Rodin Museum, 2009

Section I

A Search for Cause

Having Schizophrenia Is Unnecessary

A Diagrammatic Model of How Schizophrenia and Other Serious Disorders Develop

Parallels with a Common Illness

Chapter 1

Search For Cause

This work evolved out of deep compassion for individual patients and their families that suffered from the ravages of schizophrenia, depression and other serious mental and emotional disorders, year after year, with little or no help for what seemed to be intractable conditions. Life savings were spent to no avail, and entire families were devastated by the illness of one member.

As answers to some of these problems began to emerge, people began claiming they gained more understanding from my recordings than from all previous years of treatment. My concerns began to extend beyond the limited practice to the millions across our country and the multitudes around the world who had no such help.

How many suffer? Estimates range up to 1 percent worldwide suffer from schizophrenia, five times as many with depression, and more with attention deficit hyperactivity disorder (ADHD), school violence, autism, symbiosis, drug and alcohol dependence, eating disorders, bipolar disorder, borderline personality disorder, and more. Worse still, counting family members, we begin to see that upward of one billion people might hurt and suffer as a result of these infirmities.

Why should this epidemic of mental illness continue to exist in modern times? Could it be that nearly all are looking in the wrong direction for cause? In the race for the health care dollar, is it possible that understanding of cause has been missed altogether?

After more than forty years of research and investigation into the cause of serious mental and emotional disorders, I am well aware of a myriad of predisposing factors, precursors, antecedent factors, and contributing factors—as well as an even greater number of biological *results* of the disease process. It only takes one stone to start a landslide, so the results of the process *should* be far more numerous than the cause. Yet many *correlations* are not examined to distinguish between cause and effect. This could be a fatal error in the search for cause and might help explain why after so many decades of research, there remains a lack of conclusions that can be endorsed by all.

In the following pages, you will find another cause for serious mental and emotional disorders which few have ever considered. Yet this cause might apply to all schizophrenia, depression, and many other serious disorders. After careful review of this material, you might even conclude that without this cause, serious disorders are unlikely to occur.

Ideally, a clear understanding of the information presented here will lead to an improved ability to prevent such mental and emotional disorders and increase the potential for recovery among those who already struggle with them.

Research in these areas has often produced findings related to a relatively simple posttraumatic stress disorder mechanism. For that reason, we are compelled to consider that disease model. No stone must be left unturned.

There are two types of posttraumatic stress disorders: (1) the acute type that immediately leaves one rattled, and (2) the delayed type that follows after a terrifying event is pushed out of the conscious mind and remains buried for years or decades, only to surface later in a more severe form when a similar event occurs.

Some combat veterans, for example, have been so traumatized by their experience of death and destruction that the vividness of horrifying memories becomes an irrepressible tormentor. We all have some understanding of how this works. We have seen films of the horrors of war or have witnessed or experienced terrifying, life-threatening events ourselves; and we can appreciate how these linger in one's mind, causing nightmares, flashbacks and intrusive thoughts, high levels of anxiety, and fears throughout each day and night. The veteran remains hyper-vigilant, jumps at the slightest sound, avoids crowds and noisy places, does not socialize, and hesitates to get close to people.

One traumatized combat veteran, for example, was having a sandwich and a beer at a local pub with a couple he knew. The couple's twelve-year-old son walked in, the veteran picked up the lad and was going to give him a friendly kiss on the forehead; but suddenly he flashed back to a twelve-year-old boy in Vietnam who approached him with a live hand grenade. Instantly his mind was back in Vietnam, and he threw the child over the bar, knocked his friend to the ground and started choking him to death. His friend's wife began kicking him in the ribs. He grabbed her by the ankles, swung her around and around, flung her over the pool table, grabbed a pool stick, splintered it on the pool table, and charged his friend with the splintered end—all in less than one minute.

His friend raced out the door and across the highway. As the veteran followed in chase, the cold air hit his face. He saw cars driving on the highway and returned to current reality. His only recollection of the event was a hallucination of asking a Vietnamese woman, in Vietnamese, to see her identification pass.

This is a case of acute posttraumatic stress disorder with an extreme *hallucinatory* flashback. It represents a step back in time to earlier combat reality and behavior. Even his chemistry, physiology, and body movements matched those of the earlier time. He was strictly in a survival mode—which is highly adaptive for future combat. It enables the person to shift to autopilot and instantly respond to an attack, but it is maladaptive for social interaction.

This veteran decided never to drink beer again. Abusive substances serve as "grease in the mechanism" and facilitate a shift to the earlier time.

This whole process is just a survival mechanism. In the wild, if a gazelle escapes the attack of a lion, the next time a lion attacks, it had better do exactly what it did the first time in order to escape once more. This survival mechanism is inborn into all species. One morning, I watched young cottontails playing in the yard. They were practicing a defensive maneuver, suddenly jumping up and backward and from side to side. This skill would protect them from future hawk or osprey attack—even though they had not been attacked before. Not only are all biological, chemical, and physiological mechanisms set precisely in place, but defense mechanisms are built-in as well and these allow for survival more often than not. This is a highly effective means of adapting to future danger.

Inescapable Shock

During the time that I was engaged in the study of posttraumatic stress disorders, I was asked to evaluate survivors of disasters around the world. Within a relatively short period of time, there were invitations to four continents. In one such instance, there were more than one hundred victims of an El Al Airline disaster to evaluate from a small town near Amsterdam. A Boeing 747 had demolished a ten-story apartment building, but there were many survivors.

I happened to be reviewing a phenomenon called inescapable shock at the time. In one experiment, puppies were placed on electrical mats. Some were strapped down and others were not. The ones that were not strapped down simply jumped off the mat when it was electrified. The ones that were strapped down struggled desperately until they found they could not escape, after which they just lay there and whimpered.

Later, adult dogs were placed on electrical mats, and none were strapped down. When the mats were activated, the ones that had not been strapped down previously simply jumped off the mats, but the ones that had been strapped down the first time just lay there and whimpered. In other words, they did exactly what they did the first time in order to survive once more.

In Amsterdam, there was a unique opportunity to see this same phenomenon as it occurred in people. Only, the people were able to describe what was happening to them.

Two couples shared one apartment, and one of the four was away when the disaster struck. The other three were caught in the most frightening moments of their lives. There was a huge explosion as the Boeing 747, carrying forty thousand gallons of jet fuel, crashed into the ten-story apartment building. The building shook and rocked back and forth. They tried to escape, but found that the door had jammed shut and would not open.

They exited through the balcony with flames at their heels. It was too far to jump to the ground. Scores of people were leaping out of the building from above them to avoid being consumed by flames. The three heard horrifying screams as other victims plunged past them to their deaths below. The only chance for survival for this trio was to break the partition to the next balcony so they could move farther from the rapidly advancing fire. They did this repeatedly, from balcony to balcony, until they reached an apartment through which they could exit down a darkened, smoke-filled stairway and escape.

A year later, the same two couples were living in another apartment located near an airport. The three who were traumatized could hear airplanes so far away that sometimes it was several minutes before the fourth person was able to hear them, and whenever the three heard an airplane flying low overhead, they raced to the door. But, just like the dogs that could not jump off the mat, they could not open the door! Invariably, when they tried to open the door and couldn't, the fourth person had to open the door for them.

Why couldn't they open an unlocked door?

I concluded there is an inborn survival mechanism, which mandates that in times of similar perceived danger, the victims must replicate actions associated with survival the first time in order to optimize the chance of survival once more. The above example is a human model of inescapable shock in real life. It illustrates how and why the mechanism works, and it operates in all cases of posttraumatic stress disorder. It is a highly creative means of shifting to automatic pilot and enabling an immediate response that allows for survival more often than not. In a minority of times, however, this survival mechanism is maladaptive and works against the victim.

<u>Delayed Posttraumatic Stress Disorder (PTSD)</u>

In this type of PTSD, the original trauma is automatically repressed and stored in the unconscious mind. Each time there is a flashback, nightmare, or intrusive thought, it is added to the already-stored information related to the original trauma.

We protect ourselves from unpleasant or painful thoughts by forcing them out of our conscious awareness and closing the door on them. This is an automatic process and takes place largely without our thinking about it. It is the same as the instinctive reaction of withdrawing our hand from a hot stove. It is an automatic process that causes us to block out anything that produces physical or emotional pain.

For this reason, we forget nightmares soon after they occur. We push away flashbacks and intrusive thoughts and avoid anything reminiscent of painful or terrifying experiences.

Flashbacks and nightmares are not eliminated completely from the mind; they are stored in a separate area, loosely described as part of the unconscious mind. For simplicity, let's call this area an "abscess" of the mind. It contains all our repressed thoughts related to the trauma. The partition that contains them and keeps them out of conscious awareness is the "wall" of the abscess. The enormous force of repression accumulates, layer upon layer, year after year, to form this defensive wall.

In such cases, the person cannot return to full health. Instead, he or she becomes more distant, does not socialize, and avoids anything reminiscent of the original trauma. Keeping the original trauma in check also requires a massive amount of emotional energy.

Then one day, years or even decades after the trauma, an event occurs which is so intense and similar to the initial terrifying experience that it pierces the defense wall and stirs the unconscious material in the "abscess" of the mind. This is followed by a volcanic eruption and surfacing of the original trauma and all that it has become in the unconscious mind. The "eruption," or surfacing of the walled-off/repressed material, announces the beginning of *delayed* posttraumatic stress disorder. The graphs in chapter 3 illustrate how the "abscess of the mind" and the "wall" of the abscess are formed.

Delayed posttraumatic stress disorder surfaces sometimes many years after the original trauma. Until recently, the longest delay I had ever seen occurred in a man who was drafted into the army in 1944 while not fully recovered from meningitis.

His infirm state left him feeling quite vulnerable because he knew he did not have full control of his faculties. When asked to crawl under live machine-gun fire during basic training, he was terrified because he knew he would not be able to keep from standing up. A sergeant helped by going through the course with him and holding him down. He was so terrified that he developed angioneurotic edema, a condition in which his lips and throat swelled. It was so severe that he had to force his fingers down his throat in order to breathe.

Upon discharge from service, he married and found work in a stock brokerage firm until one day, forty-four years later, he was in a car crash, was rushed to a hospital, and placed in an MRI scanner. As soon as he heard the loud clicking sound of the scanner and was told not to move, he began hallucinating tracer bullets flying overhead—with eyes open and with eyes closed. Even the angioneurotic edema returned, causing him to thrust his fingers down his throat once more in order to breathe. From that point forward, he was 100 percent disabled with delayed posttraumatic stress disorder.

In the year 2001, a bank executive topped the veteran's record for length of delay in delayed posttraumatic stress disorder. This man's wife reported a particularly strange behavior in him. He would awaken five minutes after falling asleep, go directly to the refrigerator to eat something sweet, return to bed, and repeat this throughout the night. In the course of one year, he gained nearly one hundred pounds.

History revealed that he had a successful knee replacement and was happy with the results; but one year later, he fell and tore his knee badly, destroying the repair. He became scared of more operations, but had to endure one after another. This caused great fear, stress, and anxiety; and he thought he might lose his leg. The strange behavior and the hundred-pound weight gain started after he became fearful of more operations and losing his leg.

I commented that his awakening, putting something in his mouth, and returning to sleep is similar to the pattern of infants when they awaken, cry, and the mother puts something in their mouth. He noted that when he was born, fifty-five years earlier, his country was in civil war. Babies, being sensitive to the fears of the mother, often awaken with anxiety and cry. Ordinarily, a mother places something in the baby's mouth, and it is comforted. This is what was happening. Fear of operations returned him to the original fear, causing him to awaken throughout the night; and each time, he followed the earlier pattern of putting something in his mouth to fall asleep.

This remarkable example illustrates three things:

1. The delay can be more than half a century.
2. It can be limited to a very narrow band of feelings, reality, and behavior.
3. Its origin can be from early infancy, long prior to conscious memory.

The following chapters will demonstrate how schizophrenia closely parallels this *delayed* posttraumatic stress disorder pattern. Only, it is delayed posttraumatic stress disorder from infancy, and the symptoms more closely match the reality and behavior of the infant. The original trauma usually is not even recognized as being traumatic, and few associate the resultant behavior as belonging to an infant in the first two years of life.

Chapter 2

Having Schizophrenia Is Unnecessary

Despite the countless billions spent searching for the root cause of schizophrenia, no one, to my knowledge, has found a cause that applies to *all* schizophrenia. Nor has anyone found a cause *without which* schizophrenia cannot occur.

Imagine the frustration and discouragement of the patient who has searched for years and decades for what causes the delusional ideas to surface, over and over again, and still does not have a clue as to why this happens. And without understanding the cause, what can the patient do to prevent it from recurring?

Worse still, even those regarded as experts in the field have not found a cause that applies to all schizophrenia, and a cause without which schizophrenia cannot occur.

Those studying biochemical change have made innumerable discoveries that have led some to proclaim that schizophrenia is a chemical imbalance. There *is* a chemical imbalance indeed, but *nowhere* is there proof that this is cause instead of result of a psychological process.

Others study changes in brain structure, from minute cellular detail to gross structural change, and they indeed have made many amazing discoveries; but once more, there is *nothing* that proves this is cause instead of result of the disease process. Nonetheless, many who follow the discovery of these changes have declared schizophrenia is a *brain* disease.

Still others lump the findings together and call schizophrenia a neurobiological disorder. This is more than just declaring that neurobiological changes have been found. It goes one step further and implies that neurobiological change is the cause. Indeed, some take each new neurobiological discovery as encouragement that we are getting closer to finding *the* neurobiological cause.

This is not meant to be a criticism of the sincerity and integrity of the men and women conducting the studies. It is an observation that the enormous funding of research efforts has failed to make a crucial and verifiable distinction between cause and effect in cases of schizophrenia. It is an observation that the billions of research dollars might be spent looking *only* in the wrong direction for root cause. Indeed, the massive search for neurobiological cause might instead be a search downstream for the leak in the dam, measuring the biological results of the disease process and never addressing cause.

In the ordinary course of events, modern research institutions enjoy receiving all data supportive of their efforts. When new information presented contradicts entrenched beliefs, however, the initial reaction is often one of doubt and skepticism. Because of this barrier, serious and potentially valuable research data is blocked at the very point where it should be examined.

Science is open exploration. When critically important data is blocked, this can make it virtually impossible to identify cause; and without the identification of cause, there can be no prevention. Furthermore, without understanding the cause, mechanisms, precipitating and perpetuating factors, effective treatment is markedly compromised if not precluded altogether.

Another branch of research has spent billions of dollars in efforts to find a *genetic* cause of schizophrenia. This has resulted in more than half of the chromosomes being implicated in one study or another.

Nonetheless, only a small minority of schizophrenic patients has a first-degree relative with the disorder; and with half or more of them, the cause might be familial instead of hereditary.

In 1996 I published a textbook with Dr. Lance Wright, entitled *Delayed Posttraumatic Stress Disorders from Infancy: The Two Trauma Mechanism*, and in the literature review section I cite several errors in conclusions derived from genetic studies. For example, hereditary and familial factors are combined and counted as genetic. For me, this is not acceptable science because it lacks precision. It is like having a bushel of apples and oranges and calling them apples.

Perhaps the reason why such data is easily accepted is because the spectacular space-age technology used is so impressive that it thwarts even the *thought* of challenge. Yet hidden behind this cloak of science are many errors, and the ones I have found point in the direction of making data appear more significant than it actually is.

I have no attachment to any particular result, and the geneticists are welcome to whatever they prove. I strongly suspect there is some degree of genetic predisposition, but from the research findings I have reviewed, it is not possible to reliably determine a true percentage contribution made by that predisposition. In my opinion, genetic research is a search upstream for the leak in the dam, measuring tributaries of genetic predisposition and never addressing primary cause. Geneticists themselves do not claim they have found something that applies to all schizophrenia, and without which, schizophrenia cannot occur.

Nonetheless, as a result of the billions spent and the huge publicity this has engendered, many proclaim schizophrenia is a hereditary condition.

So thus far, while patients have not been given a clear explanation of cause and mechanisms, they have been provided a series of pronouncements, including: "It's a chemical imbalance," "It's a brain disease," "It's a neurobiological disorder," "It's hereditary," "It's a biopsychosocial disorder," or "It's many diseases with many causes." These labels are not helpful in any way; instead they are misleading. In fact, they are even more misleading because each statement is backed with billions of dollars of research and mountains of peer-reviewed literature, which makes them appear authoritative and irrefutable.

Given this as background, it is easy to understand why patients find great relief when finally they are given a clear understanding of root cause and mechanism for their illness—especially when this matches their own symptoms and life history.

In the 1981 *Schizophrenia and the McKenzie Method* audiocassette tapes, many of those responding to the questionnaire proclaimed they received more understanding from the tapes than from all previous years of treatment.

Why should this be so?

It is probably because few seem to understand enough to explain anything to the patient about how the mind works. Interest in psychological mechanisms has taken a back seat to neurobiological change, and relatively few continue to explore the workings of the mind.

Meanwhile, mental health professionals have been overwhelmed with the vast number of scientific studies, and they are awestruck with the endless volumes of peer-reviewed literature. They also are impressed with the tacit *acceptance* of current research, by virtue of enormous funding for such projects through the National Institute of Mental Health (NIMH). The mere fact that institutions receive large funding serves to validate their conclusions, including those that are flawed. The massive amount of scientific information is more than many therapists can process; and too often, they throw up their arms and say, "It's a chemical imbalance" or "It's a brain disease" or "It's a biopsychosocial disorder," depending on which section of the mountain they have chosen to climb.

What most do not realize is that all these findings might more likely pertain to the *results* of the disease process or represent minor predispositions or minor contributory factors and never truly address the actual root cause. The ultimate authority, in which they have placed their trust, could be just searching in the wrong direction for the primary cause.

I have found that when a patient is provided a clear understanding of the disorder and is able to follow the primary treatment recommendations, then psychotherapy becomes highly effective—with or without medication. In fact, medicine most often has to be reduced or eliminated altogether, because as patients recover it makes them far too drowsy.

It is not surprising that many who just listened to my audio recordings reported gaining more benefit and understanding than from all previous years of therapy. For a majority of patients, it might have been the first time they were given *any* understanding of the nature of their problem. This would explain why it comes as a great relief to them to finally know, in understandable terms, why they experienced the strange things they did. Not only do they *know,* but they also see a clear path to recovery, and recurrences are very unlikely as long as they adhere to the primary treatment protocol.

Part II: Simple Concepts Everyone Understands

We already described posttraumatic stress disorder, and this is a good place to start. Everyone understands why a veteran, ten or twenty years after the war, upon hearing a sharp sudden loud noise, instantly dives for cover or takes some other defensive measure as though he were back in combat once more.

This is simple. Although he knows where he is and knows that it is not wartime, suddenly he experiences being in another place at another time and fighting for his life. Even his chemistry and physiology change as his adrenal glands pump adrenaline into his bloodstream, his heart beats faster, he breathes harder, his pupils dilate, his hands and feet perspire, his senses are on high alert, and he scans the perimeter for danger.

What does this have to do with schizophrenia?

<u>The Posttraumatic Stress Disorder Mechanism for Schizophrenia
And How It Was Discovered</u>

The first clue came during a child psychoanalytic training class with Dr. Margaret Mahler in 1966 when she said the origin of childhood schizophrenia is in the first eighteen months of life.

Dr. Margaret Mahler is considered by many to be the foremost child psychoanalyst of the twentieth century, so her words warrant close attention.

Curious about her observation, I checked my then-current adult patient population and noted that half a dozen of my adult schizophrenic patients had a sibling about one and a half years younger—and as many of my nonpsychotic depressed patients had a sibling about two and a half years younger, and in no instance in that small patient population was this reversed.

The mutual exclusivity of the two groups, in that small patent population, is one over two to the twelfth power or one chance in 4,096 by chance alone.

Whoooa! That is worth studying. Was this just a coincidence?

<u>Birth of a sibling is only one out of thousands of infant traumas,</u> but it is very common, provides lots of data, is upsetting to many infants—and more

importantly, the exact age of the older child when the younger is born is known and recorded.

Certainly, this is no one's fault, and no one is to blame. It is a matter of an unfortunate set of circumstances at a critical stage of development, and no one would think that such an event could set the stage for the later development of a serious disorder.

Let's explore this a little further.

<u>Identifying the Age of Origin of Schizophrenia</u>

In 1966, I began to check all new patients who had serious mental and emotional disorders for this one early event—even though I knew this event was not the sole cause of all mental illness. But since the event had a known date of occurrence, it revealed something special.

As I began to study this one event, I noted that patients with schizophrenia, who had a sibling fourteen months younger, were categorically different from those with a sibling sixteen months younger; and these differed from those with a sibling eighteen months younger.

This was amazing. Soon I could determine clinically the age at birth of the next sibling, and this was accurate to the month more often than it was off by a month. This really is a broad range when we consider that it is thirty days either side of the estimate and that the rate of development between twelve and twenty-four months is very rapid. Furthermore, I had identified five parameters with which to make the determination.

I had identified age-of-origin specific reality, age-of-origin specific behavior, age-of-origin specific feelings, age-of-origin specific body movements, and age-of-origin specific level of affective expression—each of which matched the age in months of the patient when the sibling was born! So the age at birth of a sibling became *symptom defining*.

For example, a lady called on the telephone and said, "Hi, I have serotonin deficiency with a touch of paranoia," to which I replied, "Do you also have a brother or sister one year nine months younger?" Stunned, she said, "My brother is one year and nine months younger. How did you know?"

This deduction was simple because earlier I had discovered that the age *range*-of-origin of paranoid thought was mostly between twelve and twenty-one months, and the age range-of-origin of psychotic depression is mostly twenty-one to twenty-four months; so I had two parameters that met at twenty-one months, or one year and nine months.

Another lady walked into my office and greeted me, "Hi. I'm Mary. I've had schizophrenia for twelve years," to which I replied, "No you haven't. You have schizoaffective disorder. The age of origin of schizophrenia is mostly in the first eighteen months of life, and something happened to you at twenty months."

Before the session was over, I told her that the most frequent cause of her condition—in her generation when mothers spent five days in the hospital following delivery—was birth of a sibling. It was then we learned that her brother was twenty months younger. This was an easy determination because I never had met a person who had such warmth and full range of emotion and whose original symptom-defining trauma was less than twenty months. At the same time, she identified herself as having a disorder that was serious enough to be called schizophrenia for the previous twelve years. So I surmised that the origin of her disorder had to be no more than, and no less than, twenty months.

Later in this book, you will be given an opportunity to test yourself on a few clinical cases and see if you can do this too. You probably can. It's easy once you understand.

<u>Identifying the Other Traumas</u>

When I was able to identify the age of origin, based on using the birth-of-a-sibling trauma as my measuring stick, I then was able to identify other events that led to this dreaded infirmity. This was possible because I only had to search one particular month during infancy to see if anything significant had occurred during that time.

For example, in 1997, a man asked me to evaluate his son who was caught breaking into apartments. He would break in and eat all the ice cream. I told the man that something happened to his son when he was just eighteen months old. The man said no, nothing happened. I insisted that it did and he insisted that it didn't. Finally, I said, "Something happened to cause his mother to be *extremely* upset when he was just eighteen months old, and if you can't tell me, I might not be able to testify."

Tears streaked down his cheeks as he realized. It was exactly eighteen months. He knew because it happened at a New Year's party. He had an affair, his wife found out, and she was going to divorce him.

This blew over, but the damage was done, and the stage was set for the later development of the disorder.

This is how I identified the other events that set the stage for the later development of the illness.

One Common Denominator

In nearly all cases of schizophrenia, where the early history was known, the original symptom-defining trauma had one common denominator. This is a relative degree of physical or emotional separation from the mother, as experienced by the infant. Examination of the traumas reveals, almost invariably, that the separation traumas are not the parents' fault. Often they are caused by accidental events that cannot be prevented and which no one would suspect could cause such severe and lasting effects.

Brain researcher Paul MacLean found that separation from the mother is the most painful of all experiences to the mammalian infant. This produces the cry response that he could interrupt only by surgically separating the mammalian from the reptilian portion of the brain.

Indeed, for as long as mammals have populated the earth, separation from mother has meant death. We have forgotten what separation felt like at age one, but it is inborn that babies can be overwhelmed by what they consider to be a threat of physical or emotional separation from mother.

The Two-Trauma Mechanism

Then I told the man, whose son was caught breaking into apartments and eating all the ice cream, that in order for his son to have the breakdown at that time, there had to be a separation from some other most important person, probably a girlfriend and probably a couple of months prior to the appearance of his bizarre symptoms. He confirmed this, saying that his son's girlfriend had moved away two months before the strange behavior began.

In nearly every case of schizophrenia that I analyzed, it was a separation trauma in the present that precipitated the *initial* return to the separation trauma in the distant past.

This is the two-trauma mechanism: A trauma in the present, which is sufficiently intense and similar to a trauma in the distant past, can activate that original trauma and all that it has become in the unconscious mind.

With delayed posttraumatic stress disorder, the initial symptom-precipitating trauma always matches in some way the original symptom-defining trauma. In schizophrenia, since the original symptom-defining trauma is a separation from mother, the initial symptom-precipitating trauma also must be a rejection or separation from some other "most important person."

In each psychosis I analyzed, where the history was known, not only did the early separation trauma occur at the expected age, but also the *initial onset* was precipitated by another important separation—whether real, imagined, anticipated, or implied.

Sounds familiar? In delayed posttraumatic stress disorder from combat, the veteran has his initial flashback associated with a loud noise or some other terrifying element of war.

This two-trauma mechanism operates in all delayed posttraumatic stress disorders.

<u>Other Infant Traumas</u>

Over the last forty years, I identified countless other early traumas. For example, I knew a family whose barn burned down, killing all the cows. The cows were their source of income, and the mother was very fond of each one of them. Unfortunately, not only was she grieving over the loss of the animals she loved and worrying about the loss of their livelihood, but more importantly, her attention was drawn away from her eighteen-month-old baby, producing an emotional separation trauma. Twenty years later when a girlfriend rejected him, he shifted to the eighteen-month reality and met full criteria for schizophrenia.

When I saw the movie *A Beautiful Mind*, I e-mailed John Nash and said, "Based on the facts as presented in the movie, it is my opinion that the origin of your disorder is close to fifteen months." I knew it was not quite within the more bizarre thirteen-to-fifteen-month age range-of-origin, but it was close. Indeed, it proved to be fifteen and a half months. When he was fifteen months old, the stock market was 400, and when he was sixteen months old in October 1929, it was 200. Mothers, who were focused on their babies, suddenly focused on survival. I previously had identified this particular trauma in the textbook *Delayed Posttraumatic Stress Disorders from Infancy: The Two Trauma Mechanism*.

It Is Not the Parents' Fault

All original traumas had one common denominator, which is a relative degree of physical or emotional separation from the mother, as experienced by the baby. These are not terrible rejections or anything of the kind. Usually they represent an unfortunate set of circumstances at a critical stage of development. In fact, the better the relationship with the mother and the better the bonding, the more upsetting it is when separation occurs. In 1945, Rene Spitz reported that half of the infants in fondling homes, who had experienced early separation from mother, died by age two in spite of good medical care. Those who had *good* bonding in the first four to six months prior to separation, were more severely affected.

Why should separation be as terrifying to a baby as war trauma to a soldier? This makes no sense until we realize that *for as long as mammals have populated the earth, separation from mother has meant death.*

The Purpose of Schizophrenia

The only purpose I have found for schizophrenia is survival, but in schizophrenia, the survival mechanism is maladaptive.

This same survival mechanism applies in all cases of posttraumatic stress disorder, and in many situations, it is maladaptive.

For the veteran, it is highly adaptive for future combat. It is not necessary to think about what to do. Instantly, he moves into "automatic pilot" and takes defensive action.

This bypasses thought processes. It is a knee-jerk response, like touching a hot stove, and it counts for survival more often than not. I recall a combat veteran who, on a foggy night in Philadelphia, was approached by a man wearing a trench coat and asking for a light. As the man started to pull a shotgun out from under his coat, the veteran instantly grabbed it, jerked it out of his hands, struck him between the eyes with the butt of the gun, threw the gun across the street, and ran—all in about three seconds. Combat veterans can be very dangerous when confronted or startled because they automatically return to previous life-and-death, hand-to-hand combat with little provocation. This is highly adaptive for future combat, but maladaptive for watching war movies in a theater.

A similar phenomenon occurs when police officers experience life-and-death confrontations by persons wielding deadly weapons. Home videos of their overreactions to benign situations make the officers appear to go berserk without due cause. Their "due cause" belongs to a previous life-and-death struggle, combined with a primordial survival instinct that is to rip, tear, bite, claw until there is no sign of life in the other individual.

Since survival is such a strong behavioral drive, a perceived threat to one's survival is the driving force behind any posttraumatic stress disorder—whether it is posttraumatic stress disorder from infancy (schizophrenia) or posttraumatic stress disorder from war.

This survival mechanism not only protects us in case the same event should occur again, but it even protects us from experiencing the painful thoughts and feelings (through repression) and protects us from being in the same danger situation again (through the avoidance phenomena).

Prevention

We cannot prevent the next sibling from arriving at a critical age for the older child, and we cannot prevent the stock market from crashing or the house from burning down, but we can recognize the impact on the baby and make that our primary focus, bringing additional comfort to the baby at those times. Greater recognition and knowledge of what to do will dramatically reduce the incidence of mental and emotional disorders.

As we continue to learn more about the origin and mechanisms of serious mental and emotional disorders and identify more of the innocent little traumas to babies which no one recognizes, we will be able to prevent or modify those original traumas and thereby reduce or eliminate the disorders in future generations.

As you read on, you also will learn how to prevent a first psychotic or major depressive episode from occurring in a vulnerable child, and you will learn new methods of preventing a recurrence among those who already have developed a serious disorder.

Chapter 3

Diagrams of Schizophrenia and Delayed Posttraumatic Stress Disorder from Adult Life

One picture is worth a thousand words. For clarity, I therefore will illustrate schizophrenia in diagrammatic form and compare it to delayed posttraumatic stress disorder from adult life. In this way, we can see, point by point, that schizophrenia meets criteria for delayed posttraumatic stress disorder.

In psychiatry, there is a description and a label for nearly everything, but often with a little or no understanding how and why the phenomenon occurs.

I re-define <u>schizophrenia</u> as the co-existence of two minds in one skull: the mind and brain of the adult combined with the mind and brain of the troubled infant. The <u>positive symptoms</u> are largely the delusions, hallucinations, excitement and bizarre behavior, and the <u>negative symptoms</u> are the numbing of affect, social withdrawal and avoidance phenomena.

The diagrams illustrate, for the first time, the derivation of the precursors of schizophrenia and the derivation of the negative symptoms of schizophrenia. These correspond precisely with the numbing of affect, social withdrawal and avoidance phenomena found in delayed PTSD from adult life.

The diagrams also show the derivation of acute positive symptoms of schizophrenia and how this matches the derivation of acute positive symptoms of delayed PTSD from adult life.

We see how schizophrenia requires a trauma in the first two years of life, coupled with a similar trauma years or decades later to activate it—and we see how this same two-trauma mechanism operates in delayed PTSD from adult life.

In the charts that follow, you will find an initial symptom-defining trauma that occurs at a precise chronological age, identified on the chart as point A.

As flashbacks, nightmares and intrusive thoughts occur, they continue to connect with the age-of-origin-specific original trauma in the unconscious mind. If the original trauma occurs at age three hundred sixty-five days, then each flashback, nightmare and intrusive thought connects to the traumatic experience in the mind and brain of the infant at that precise age. Gradually these thoughts, as they accumulate year after year, become a growing "abscess" of the mind.

With each new inclusion into the "abscess" of the mind, there is a shield of repression that restrains it and keeps it out of conscious awareness. This shield becomes the "wall" of the abscess, and *as the "abscess" of the mind grows, the "wall" of the abscess thickens.*

Eventually, years or decades later, there is an initial *symptom-precipitating trauma* at point B, which is *sufficiently intense and similar* to the original symptom-defining trauma at point A, that it pierces the defensive wall and activates the original trauma and all that it has become in the unconscious mind. This produces a volcanic eruption and a surfacing of the unconscious material that had been restrained. It represents a *partial* return to the earlier mind/brain/reality/feelings/behavior/chemistry/physiology/body movements/ level of affective expression and neuroanatomic sites in the brain that were active and developing at the precise time of the original trauma. In schizophrenia, this is heralded as the appearance of acute positive symptoms.

If the trauma is a war experience from adult life, then the person shifts to combat reality and behavior. This is delayed posttraumatic stress disorder from adult life, and it is accompanied by the changes in chemistry and physiology associated with the terrifying events of war. Since this occurred in adult life, the activity remains largely in the adult developmental regions of brain.

The defensive wall, in the traumatized adult, is recognized clinically as numbing of affect, social withdrawal, amnesia, and avoidance of anything reminiscent of war. In schizophrenia, prior to the onset of acute illness at point B, this defensive wall is called the <u>precursors of schizophrenia</u>. It is the same as the defensive wall in delayed posttraumatic stress disorder from adult life, only it is the child who is shy, timid, does not socialize, does not participate in rough sports, and does *nothing* to stir the sleeping giant inside the abscess of the mind.

After the symptom-precipitating trauma at point B, the same defensive wall in schizophrenia changes names and is called the <u>negative symptoms</u> of schizophrenia.

The original symptom-defining trauma at point A is the precursor of the precursors of schizophrenia.

Once the defensive wall is compromised at point B, it remains less intact and acute illnesses can recur with little further provocation.

So let us begin with the diagrams for clarity. We will simply put the above explanations into diagrammatic form.

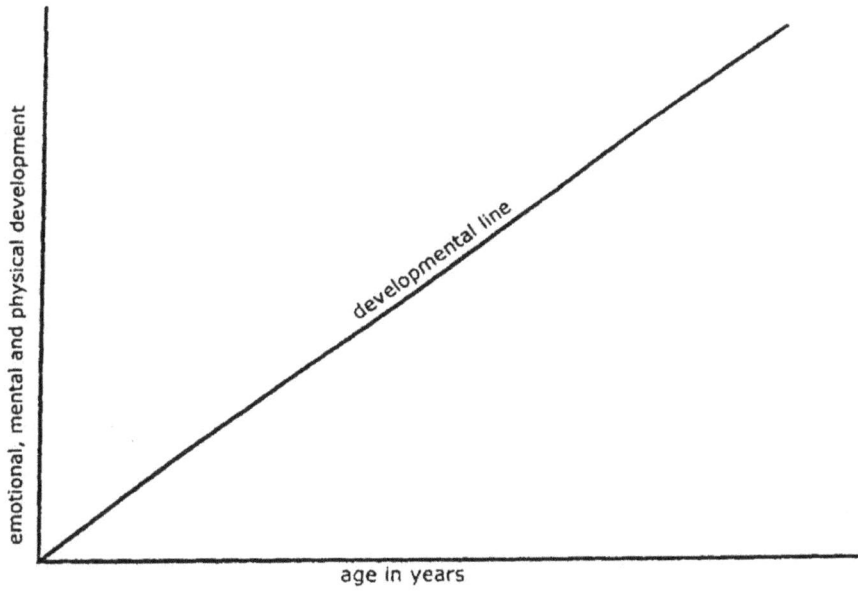

The horizontal line is age in years. The vertical line represents mental, emotional, and physical development. *The diagonal line is the developmental line and represents how developed a person is at any particular age.*

The remainder of this chapter is for those who want a more in-depth understanding of the mental process.

The charts show:

1. the original symptom-defining trauma,
2. the *accumulation* of flashbacks, nightmares and intrusive thoughts over the years, described as a growing *abscess* of the unconscious mind,
3. the accumulation of a *wall* of repression that grows with each flashback, nightmare and intrusive thought, and
4. the occurrence of a symptom-precipitating trauma later in life, which is similar to the symptom-defining trauma, and which *activates* the original traumatic experience *and all that it has become in the unconscious mind*. This can occur years or decades later, and is recognized as the onset of delayed posttraumatic stress disorder.

Results:

1. If the *original* trauma occurred during adult life, it can resurface as delayed posttraumatic stress disorder from adult life—which is what we often see in the combat veteran.
2. If the *original* trauma occurred in the first two years of life, it can become psychosis if activated later in life, i.e., the person begins to experience the reality/feelings/behavior of the infant. Depending on the age in months when the original trauma occurred, the patient can have schizophrenia, schizo-affective disorder, bipolar disorder, or psychotic depression—in that order but with some overlap.
3. If the *original* trauma occurred in the third year of life, it can become non-psychotic depression.

You absolutely do not need to study these charts—if they perplex you. But to those who study and understand them, they become amazingly clear, simple and precise. Many reviewers in our beta-test group went blank when they saw the original graphs. We have simplified the graphs since, but if this happens to you, just read on and ultimately you will understand them.

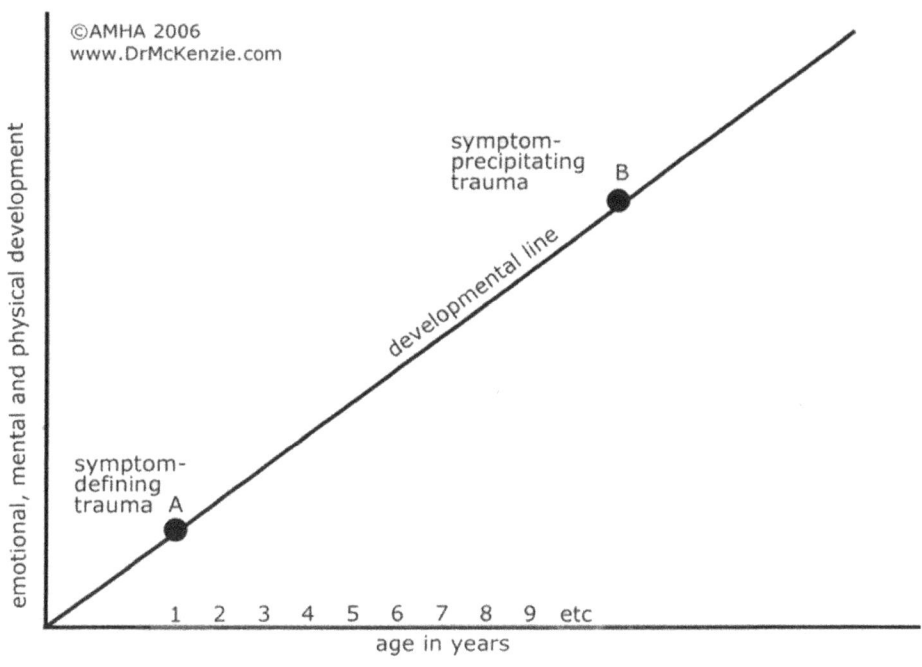

Point A on the diagram represents the original symptom-defining trauma. With schizophrenia, the symptoms are defined largely by the age in months, in the first two years of life, when the original symptom-defining trauma occurred.

Point B represents the initial symptom-precipitating trauma. If at point B you find the patient upside down in a fetal position trying to force his head through a toilet bowl, you can surmise that the symptom-defining trauma occurred right at birth. That's how precise this mechanism is.

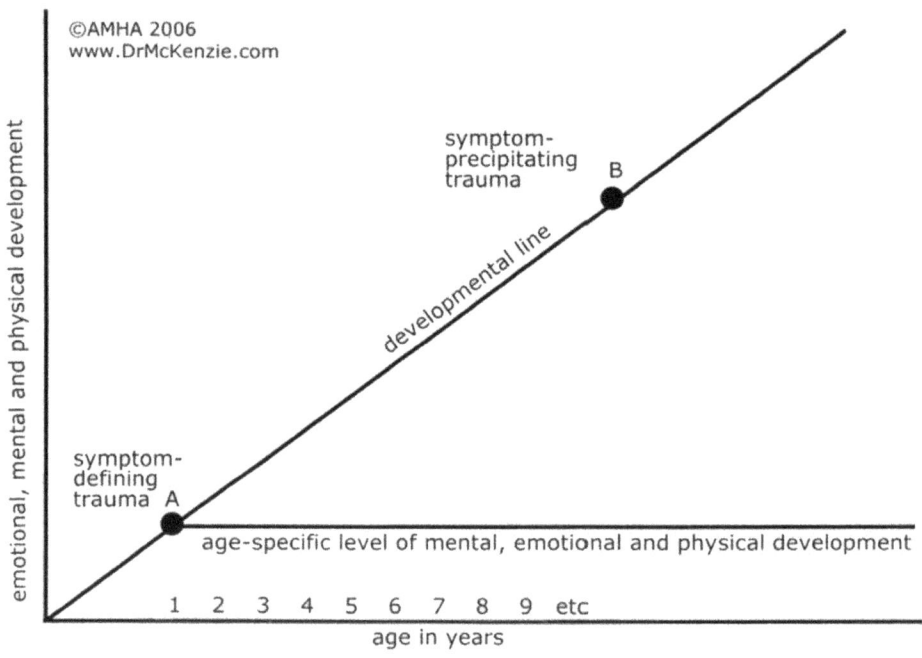

The horizontal line that starts at point A represents an age-specific level of mental, emotional, and physical development that existed at the time of the original symptom-defining trauma. *If the original trauma occurred at age one year, then it represents the one-year-old mind and brain.*

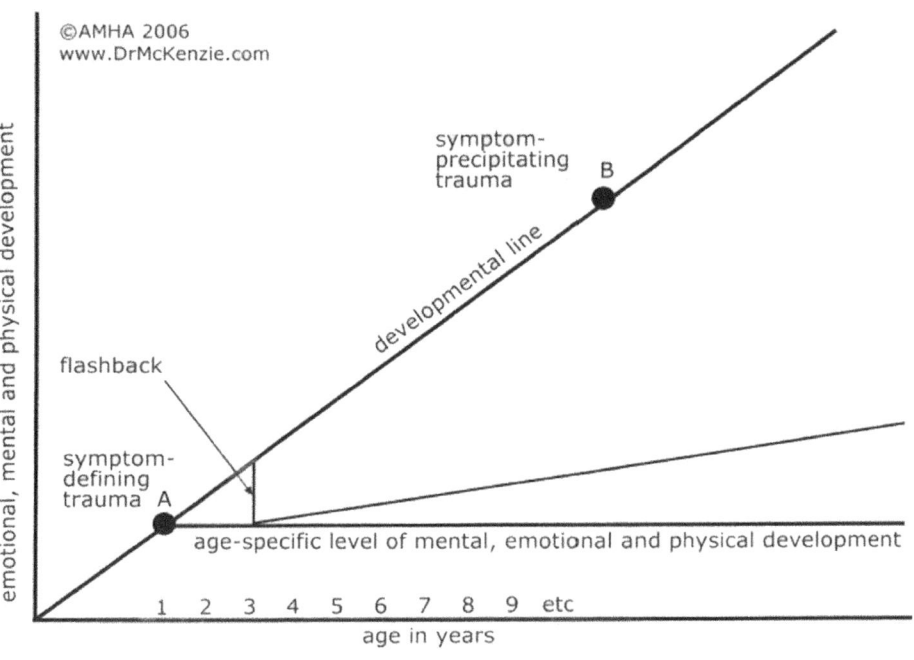

Flashback

A flashback occurs when an event causes a person to re-experience the original trauma.

It connects a present event with the trauma that is recorded in an age-specific earlier developmental region of mind and brain. Each flashback adds to that earlier developmental region of brain.

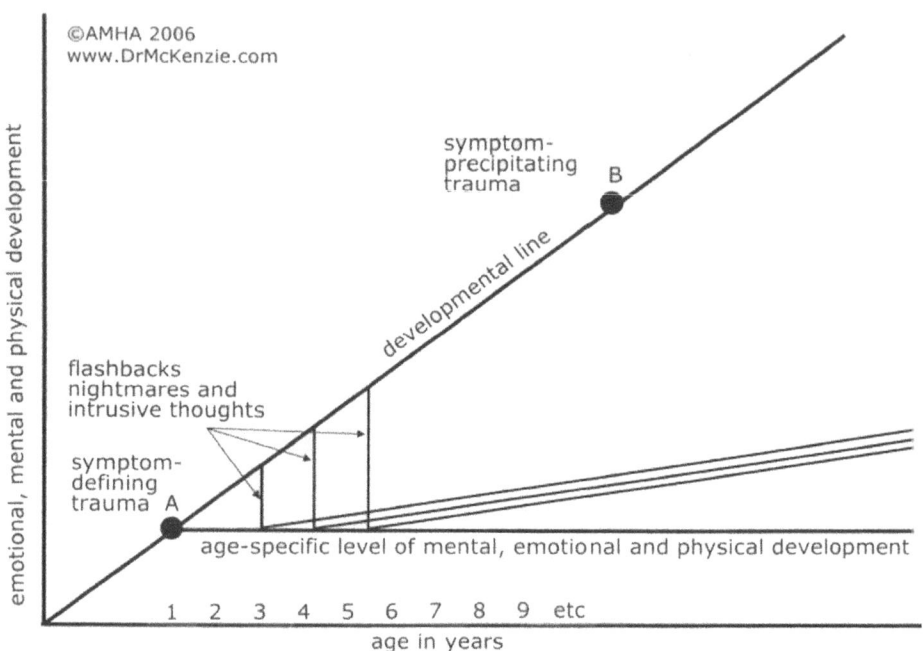

Flashbacks, Nightmares, and Intrusive Thoughts

Each flashback, nightmare and intrusive thought connects with and feeds into the original traumatic experience in the earlier part of the mind and brain.

Therefore, *if the trauma occurred at age one, then the one-year-old mind and brain experiences the trauma over and over again, year after year, with each flashback, nightmare and intrusive thought.*

Eventually, this grows into an age-of-origin specific "abscess" of the mind.

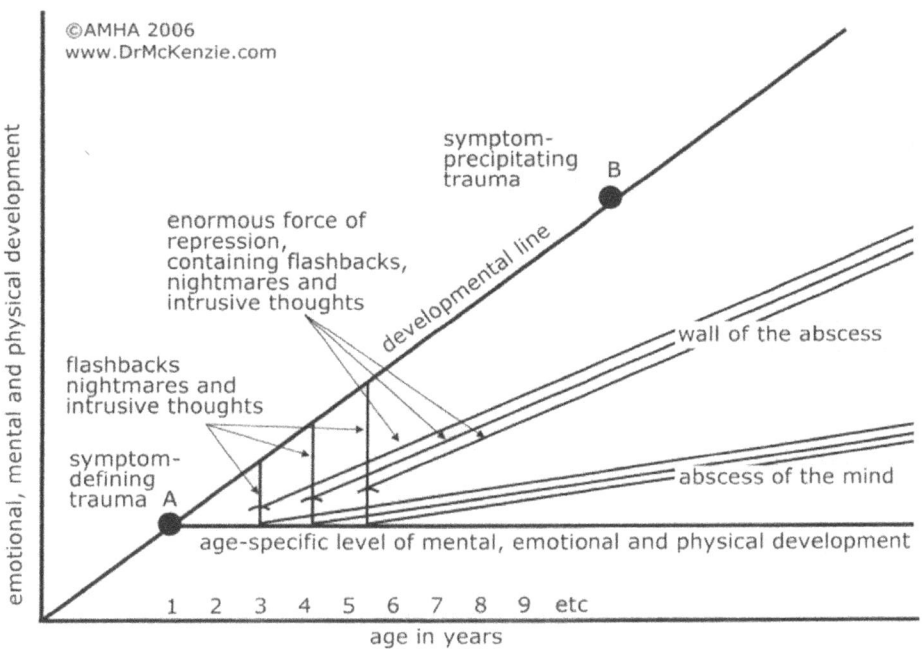

Repression: The Defensive Wall that Contains the Abscess of the Mind

Each flashback, nightmare and intrusive thought requires active repression to contain it and keep it out of the conscious mind. This is an automatic process. Dreams are quickly forgotten, flashbacks and unpleasant thoughts are pushed out of the mind. This continuing process of repression forms the defensive "wall" of the abscess, which is represented by the lines that run above the growing "abscess" of the mind.

In the diagram to the right, point A represents an original trauma, an overwhelming event.

A flashback occurs later, when something causes the person to re-experience the original, frightening event.

The flashback *connects* with this terrifying event. It doesn't matter if the flashback occurs years or decades later; it still must connect with the age-of-origin specific event. It connects to the same early point in time, the same age-specific developmental area of mind, the same region of brain where the original event was recorded.

Intrusive thoughts and nightmares do the same. Thus over the course of years, the flashbacks, nightmares and intrusive thoughts accumulate around the original point in time, the specific region of mind and brain to which the flashback pertains. If the original trauma occurred at age 21, then all flashbacks, nightmares and intrusive thoughts connect with the 21-year-old part of the mind and brain. If it occurred at age one, then all flashbacks, nightmares and intrusive thoughts connect with the one-year-old part of the mind and brain.

This becomes a growing abscess of the mind and brain. Like the original terrifying event, it also connects with the integrated network of body/mind/brain/reality/feelings/behavior/chemistry/physiology/body movements/level of affective expression and neuro-anatomic sites in the brain that were active and developing at the precise time of the original symptom-defining trauma of the earlier time.

Year after year, decade after decade, this "abscess" continues to grow in the unconscious mind.

Is this not simple? Does it not make sense? Every time one *re*-experiences an overwhelming traumatic event, it connects with the original traumatic event in the same part of the mind and brain. It stirs the same chemical and physiological reactions, and it adds to the original event.

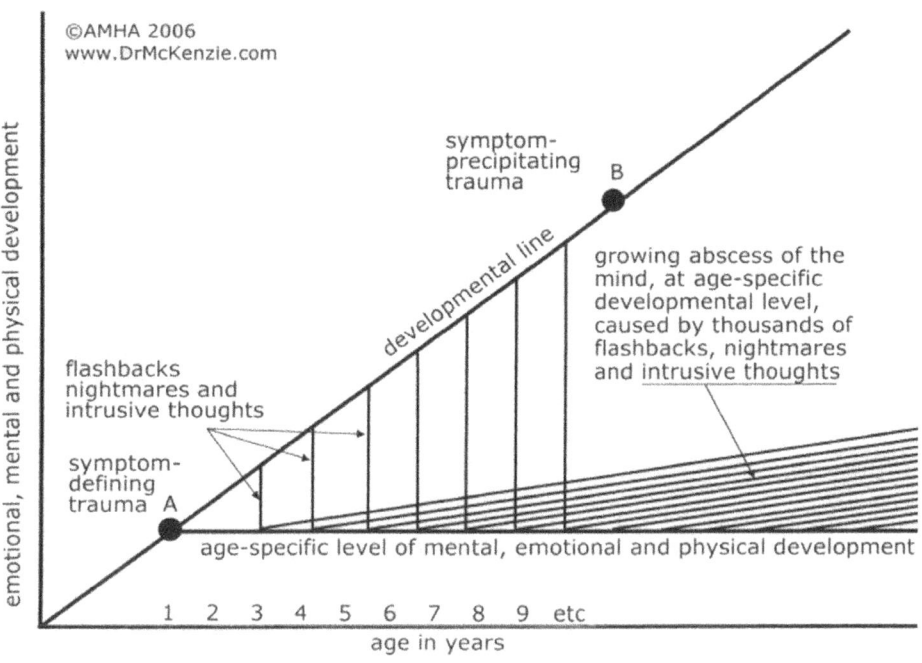

Over the course of many years, all flashbacks, nightmares and intrusive thoughts related to the original trauma, connect with and become a part of a growing abscess of the mind, as the trauma can be re-experienced many thousands of times.

Preschool children, who experienced an overwhelming separation trauma at age one, for example, literally scream when mother goes out to the store. Ordinarily this is not even recognized as a flashback.

In the diagram to the right, you see that every flashback, nightmare and intrusive thought connects with the original overwhelming trauma, forming an age-of-origin specific "abscess" of the mind.

Each flashback, nightmare and intrusive thought automatically is forced out of the conscious mind and held in the unconscious mind by an active process of repression. This becomes the "wall" of the abscess.

This unconscious process requires an enormous amount of emotional energy.

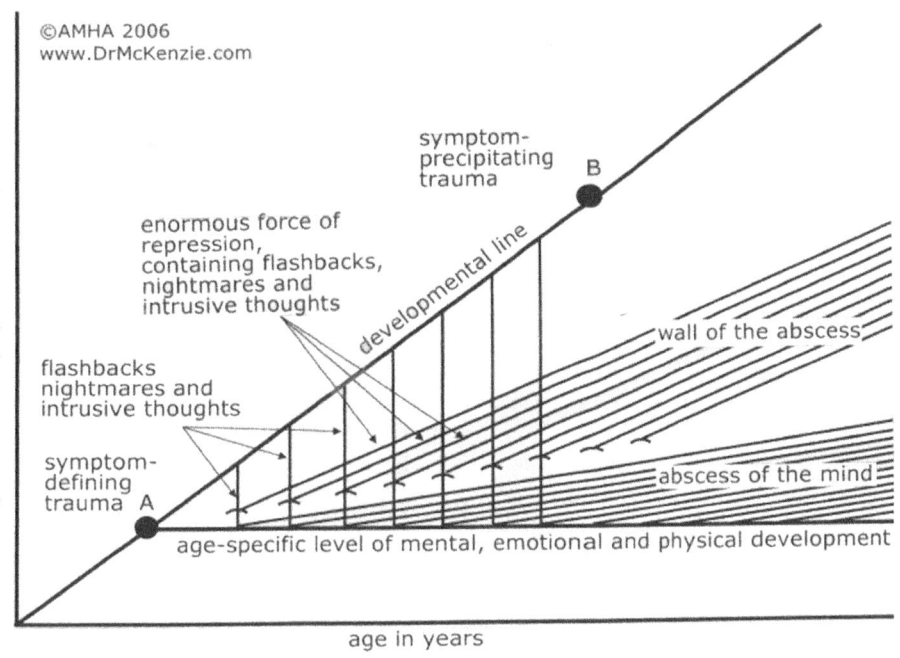

The wall of the abscess builds with each unwanted flashback, nightmare and intrusive thought, and *as the abscess grows the wall thickens.*

This abscess is what Pierre Janet, in 1886, called an isolated core nucleus of consciousness, and the diagram illustrates how it develops.

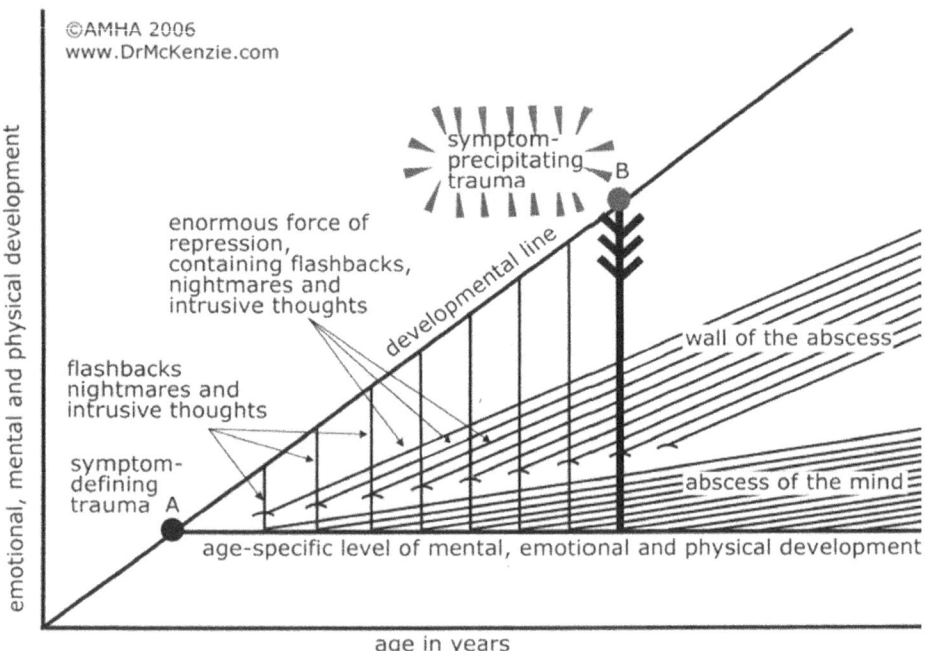

Initial Symptom-precipitating Trauma

Eventually, there is a symptom-precipitating trauma at point B, which is sufficiently intense and similar to the original symptom-defining trauma at point A, that it impacts the defensive wall.

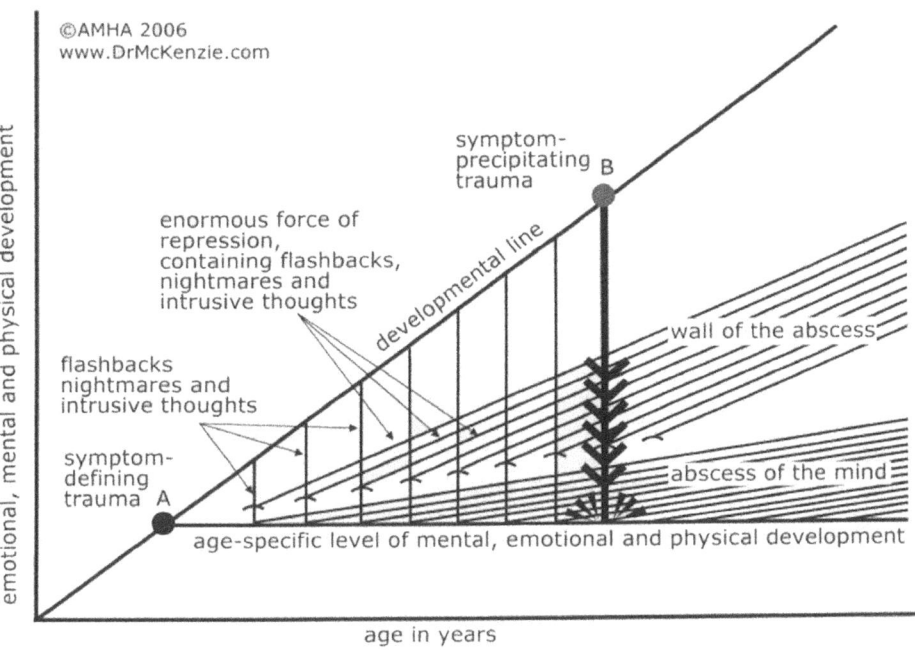

If the trauma at point B is sufficiently intense and similar to the trauma at point A, it will penetrate the defensive wall and activate the isolated core nucleus of consciousness, or the growing abscess of the mind.

Stress factors and abusive substances can serve to weaken the defensive wall and facilitate its breach.

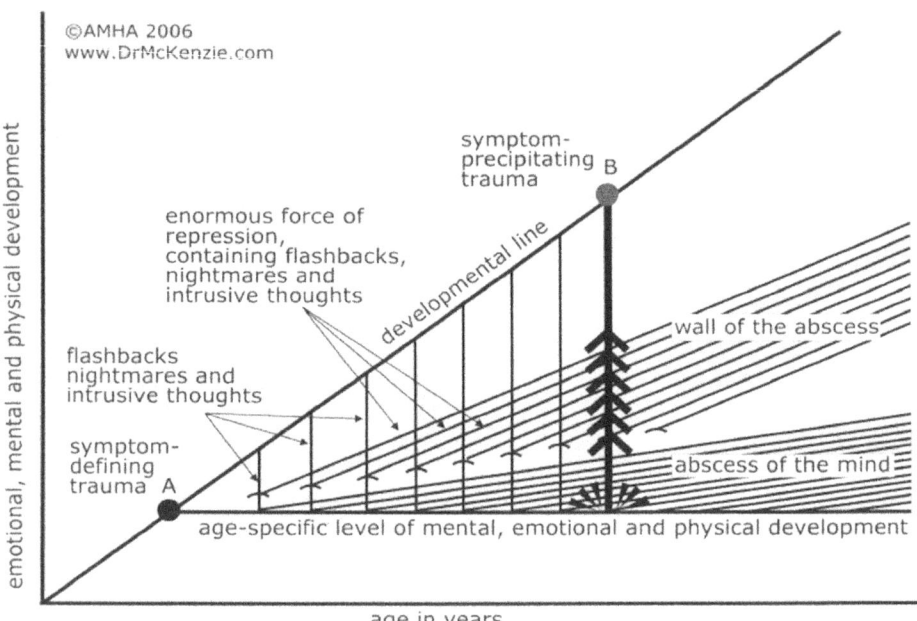

Once the nightmares, flashbacks and intrusive thoughts contained in the abscess of the mind make a sufficiently intense impact on the symptom-precipitating trauma, a powerful reaction occurs which overcomes the defensive wall of the abscess.

This is a survival mechanism, and all previous means of coping with the earlier dangers are reactivated, even though the coping mechanisms might no longer apply to the present situation and might therefore be maladaptive.

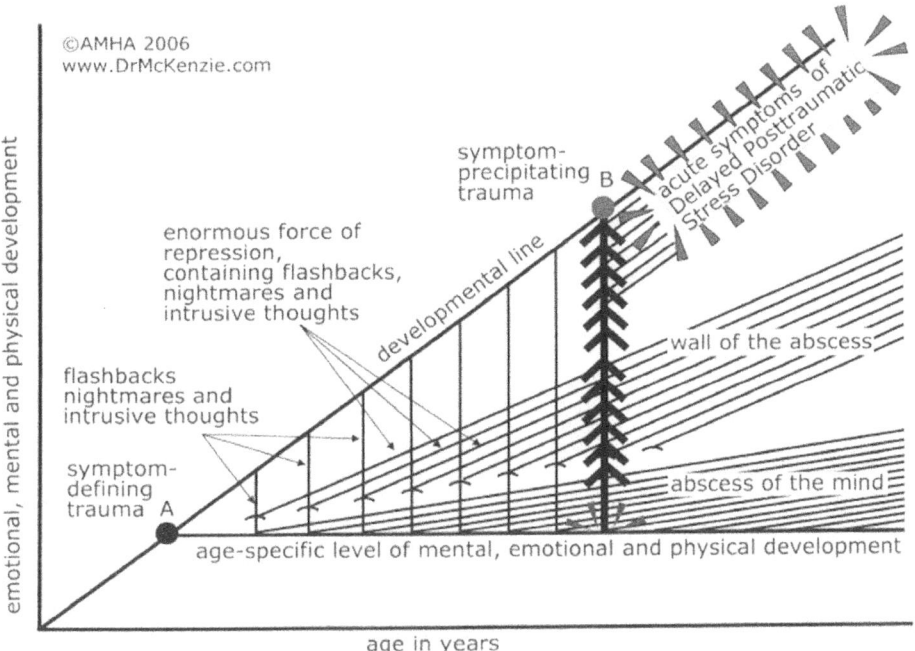

The volcanic eruption that bursts through the wall of the abscess, results in part, or all, of the growing abscess of the mind surfacing, and this is recognized as the acute positive symptoms of delayed Posttraumatic Stress Disorder.

If the symptom-defining trauma at point A is a war trauma that occurs at age eighteen *years*, then at point B, we have acute positive symptoms of delayed PTSD from adult life—with the sudden appearance of outbursts of uncontrolled aggression, hyper vigilance, and increased startle reflex.

The wall of the abscess—in the adult traumatized during war—is recognized clinically as numbing of affect, social withdrawal, amnesia, and avoidance of anything reminiscent of war.

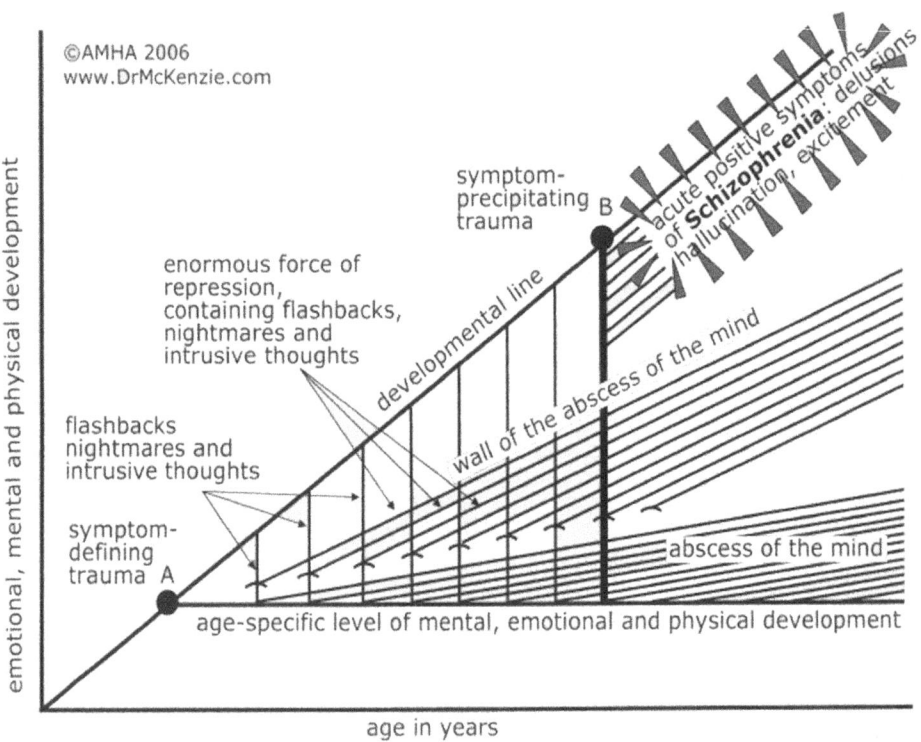

If the symptom-defining trauma at point A is a separation trauma that occurs at eighteen <u>months</u>, then at point B, we have the acute positive symptoms of schizophrenia (delusions, hallucinations, excitement).

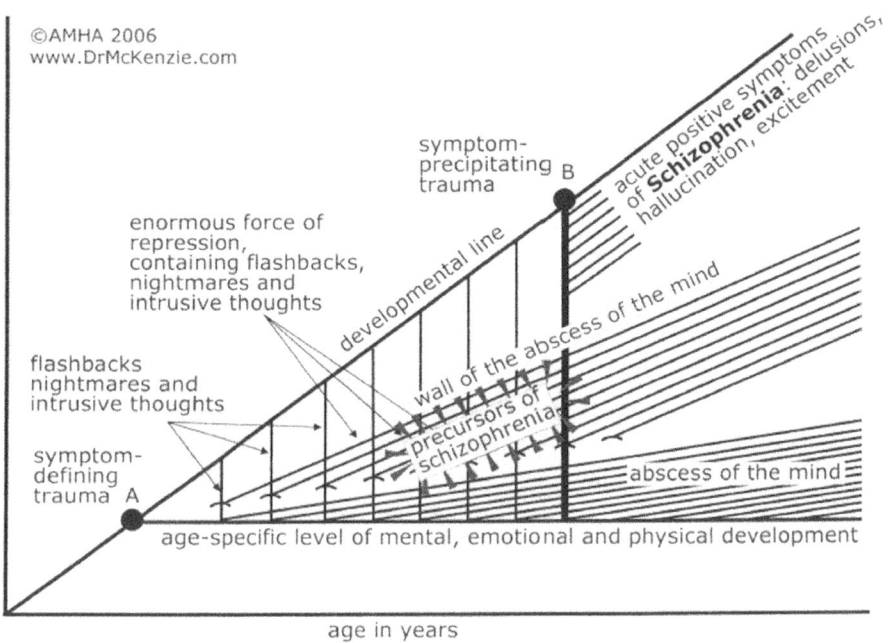

From point A to point B, the defensive wall is called the precursors of schizophrenia: This is the same wall that we have with delayed posttraumatic stress disorder from adult life, only it is the child who is shy, timid, does not socialize, does not participate in rough sports, and does nothing to stir the sleeping giant inside this abscess of the mind.

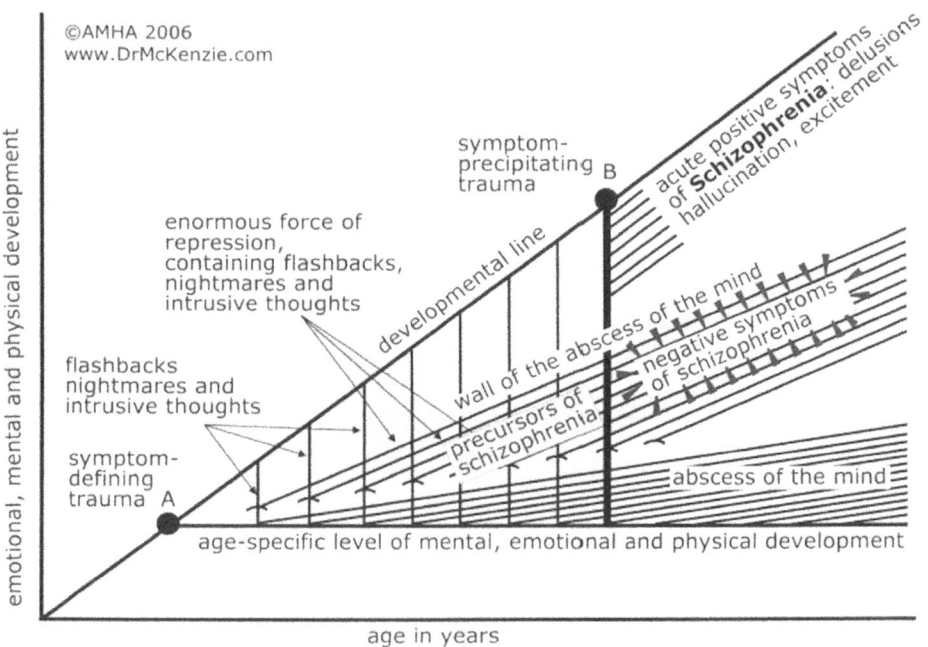

After the symptom-precipitating trauma at point B, the same defensive wall changes names and is called the negative symptoms of schizophrenia.

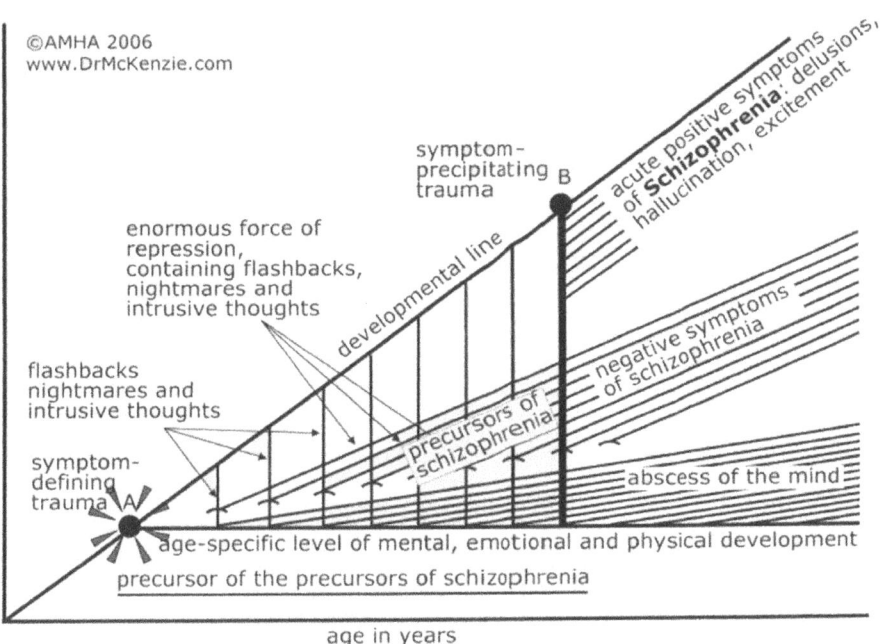

The symptom-defining trauma that occurs at point A, incidentally, is the *precursor* of the precursors of schizophrenia.

Note: Once the defensive wall is compromised at point B, the wall remains less intact and the acute illness can recur with little further provocation.

You might wish to refer back to the diagrams for clarity from time to time.

Chapter 4

Does Schizophrenia Meet the Diagnostic Criteria for Delayed Posttraumatic Stress Disorder?

If schizophrenia meets criteria for delayed posttraumatic stress disorder, as I am convinced it does, then there is an enormous benefit to worldwide recognition and acceptance of this finding because if it is so, then it means we can actually prevent schizophrenia—and for the first time!

With correct understanding, we not only can change the name from schizophrenia to delayed posttraumatic stress disorder, reducing some of the stigma associated with the condition, but far more importantly, we can prevent most schizophrenia from ever occurring.

There have been major obstacles to bringing this work forward. Schopenhauer once noted, "All truth passes through three stages: first, it is ridiculed; second, it is violently opposed; third, it is accepted as being self-evident." Hopefully, we are moving into the third stage because it is unnecessary for millions to develop schizophrenia.

Our focus must be on the next generation of families who need protection from developing schizophrenia and other serious disorders, on mothers who never would want to cause harm to the babies they love so much, and on babies who need protection from separation traumas.

The graphs in chapter 3 illustrate the derivation of the components of delayed posttraumatic stress disorder and help illustrate twelve clear and precise parallels between delayed posttraumatic stress disorder from infancy (schizophrenia) and delayed posttraumatic stress disorder from adult life. Regardless of age of origin, the original symptom-defining trauma is experienced as overwhelming and even life threatening. A subsequent trauma years or decades later can precipitate a partial return to the earlier time, with the feelings, behavior, reality, chemistry and physiology of the earlier time.

When the original trauma occurs *during the first two years of life*, a second trauma later in life can precipitate a psychosis, which is a return to the precise mental age when the first trauma occurred. The person begins experiencing the original trauma and all that it has become in the unconscious mind. When we understand this, then we realize that in the psychotic, instead of *un*reality, it is *earlier* reality we see, and instead of bizarre behavior, it is *earlier* behavior that occurs. It is extremely important to make these distinctions.

In all delayed posttraumatic stress disorder, this shift to an earlier time is the result of a survival mechanism that causes persons to go onto automatic pilot, which is helpful for future combat, but maladaptive for the veteran watching war movies in a theater and maladaptive in schizophrenia when there is a shift to infant mind/brain/reality.

<u>Recurrent Episodes</u>

Regardless of age of origin, *the defensive wall of delayed posttraumatic stress disorder is less intact after it is breached by the initial symptom-precipitating trauma*. Thus, even a mild stimulus can trigger a recurrence.

Following the first psychotic episode, *subsequent ones occur with little further provocation*. After a first major depressive episode, *there can be multiple recurrent ones*. After a first panic attack or phobia, *recurrences take place readily*; and after "crossing the invisible line" in alcoholism, all it takes is one drink to return to the infant-on-the-bottle mind/brain/reality in which the alcoholic drinks until the belly is full and passes out.

With delayed posttraumatic stress disorder from combat, after initial onset caused by the initial symptom-precipitating trauma, almost anything can trigger recurrences. Even popcorn popping in the next room might sound like machine-gun fire in the distance.

With delayed posttraumatic stress disorder from infancy, following initial onset, any loss, separation, or rejection—or even involvement with family—can precipitate acute symptoms once more.

With either delayed posttraumatic stress disorder from infancy or from adult life, there is a partial return to the entire earlier gestalt, i.e., a partial return to the earlier mind/brain/reality/feelings/behavior/chemistry/physiology/body movements/level of affective expression and neuroanatomic sites in the brain that were active and developing at the precise time of the original symptom-defining trauma. This is because the survival mechanism causes a partial return to the entire physical, mental, and emotional process that enabled the person to survive the first time.

Clinical Example of Shift to Infant Reality

Everyone recognizes when a combat veteran shifts to the terrifying reality of war, but the shift to infant reality is not as obvious. Here is an example to refresh our memory.

One young man continued to experience that people were putting poison in his drink, and this went on for years.

In actuality his drink *had* been spiked when he was a baby. His mother was very loving and caring, but periodically her husband caused her great stress, and she would turn to drinking for a few days. This produced emotional separation trauma for the baby, and during those times his drink (breast milk) *was* spiked and he *knew* it! Consequently, when he shifted to this earlier reality, he absolutely knew that someone put something in his drink. This is why it is so difficult to convince patients it is not real. They know it *is* real.

A Neurobiological Distinction Between Delayed PTSD from Infancy and Delayed PTSD from Adult Life

A major difference is that delayed posttraumatic stress disorder from infancy (schizophrenia) causes reactivation of the earlier developmental brain structures that were active and developing during the first two years of life. These are the structures that produce more dopamine and other neurotransmitters involved in the disease process, and when reactivated, they produce more. The corresponding shift of brain activity away from the later developmental brain structures results in brain atrophy, as would occur in any other area of the body that becomes less active.

This shift of brain activity, from adult brain structures to those developing during infancy, results in the vast number of biological changes that have been described in schizophrenia, and which mistakenly are identified as cause.

I have studied countless neurobiological changes and determined that all of the ones I reviewed are more likely the *result* instead of the *cause* of this psychological process. In fact, each biological change is what we should expect to find with a shift of brain activity away from the adult brain structures and into the brain structures that were active and developing at the precise time of the original symptom-defining trauma during infancy. (See Appendix)

When we find biological change that correlates with schizophrenia, ordinarily it is difficult to determine whether it is cause or result of the psychological process—but the data on 6,000 schizophrenic patients in the Finnish database and the data on 2,669 in the Danish cohort on schizophrenia correlate with a specific trauma in the first two years of life, and no one can argue in the reverse direction—i.e., no one can say that the patients had the trauma in the first two years of life because thirty years later they developed schizophrenia!

This eliminates the cause-versus-effect dilemma from the correlation.

A Multitude of Less Important Factors

After forty years of studying schizophrenia, I am aware of the many other contributing factors that become significant when surveying large populations; but with delayed posttraumatic stress disorder, *there is a one-to-one correlation with earlier trauma* because by definition, you cannot have delayed posttraumatic stress disorder without original trauma.

I also am aware of genetic predisposition, stress factors, and antecedent traumas that make the original symptom-defining trauma more intense. With schizophrenia, the antecedent traumas include second trimester factors, pre-and perinatal traumas, birth trauma, circumcision, and other less important separations. But without the symptom-defining trauma, coupled with the symptom-precipitating trauma, there is no return to the infant mind, the infant brain, the infant reality, the infant feelings, the infant behavior, the infant chemistry, the infant physiology, the infant body movements, the infant level of affective expression, and the infant neuroanatomic sites in the brain that were active and developing at the precise time of the original symptom-defining trauma in the first two years of life.

One of the antecedent factors to which boys are subjected but girls are not is circumcision—without anesthesia and without the mother present. This antecedent trauma can add significantly to the original symptom-defining trauma and probably is the reason for the earlier onset of schizophrenia in boys over girls. This trauma causes the original separation trauma to be more severe, and the more severe the original symptom-defining trauma, the sooner a subsequent trauma can come along to precipitate the initial onset of schizophrenia. This is because a mild trauma in the present can activate a severe trauma from the past, whereas it takes a severe trauma in the present to activate a mild trauma from the past. Consequently, since circumcision augments the original symptom-defining trauma, the symptom-precipitating trauma need not be as great—which means that a trauma that is sufficiently intense to precipitate initial onset of the disorder is more likely to occur sooner.

It is unlikely that others have considered these factors. The scientific appearance given by modern technology, the tacit endorsement by NIMH through the awarding large sums for such research, and the mountains of peer-reviewed journal articles by esteemed individuals at prestigious universities have blinded the eyes of many, even to incontrovertible truths, and caused most to turn away from considering trauma-related origin.

Who Has Endorsed This Work?

I cite a few commentaries by noted persons in the field to help you decide the validity of the findings in this area:

In 1984, I presented a paper in Madrid entitled "The Anatomy and Psychodynamics of Psychosis" and I sent a copy to Paul MacLean, chief of Brain Evolution and Behavior at NIMH, who had just written *The Triune Brain*. He wrote a very enthusiastic reply, proclaiming that it went beyond the child development theories of Dr. Margaret Mahler, and he concurred with where and how the schizophrenic process was taking place in the brain—and he was one of the leading brain researchers of the day.

Then Sarnoff Mednick of the University of Southern California, in 1994, wrote, "I was skeptical about Dr. McKenzie's findings, but the Finnish database on 6,000 schizophrenic patients revealed a very high level of statistical significance. We confirmed a substantially higher rate of schizophrenia among those with siblings less than two years younger."

O. Spurgeon English, one of the most respected psychoanalysts of the twentieth century, called this work the new unification theory of mental illness and wrote, "Theory is a marriage between psychological and biological, spanning the neuroses and the psychoses, from infancy to old age." He further wrote, "The findings . . . show that psychiatric illnesses are based on early trauma and follow a pattern of later activation precipitated by a major life crisis or significant stressor, and then multiple reactivations with little further provocation. This delayed posttraumatic stress disorder pattern of activation and reactivation holds true not only for schizophrenia, but also for mood disorders, anxiety disorders, psychoactive substance use disorders, eating disorders and more." And he added, "While valuable treatment concepts evolved out of the new understanding, the most powerful implications are for prevention."

Charles Figley, founding editor in chief of the *Journal of Traumatic Stress*, wrote that this work "fits like a glove with what is known about traumatic stress." He also wrote that this work "breaks ground in suggesting the role of early trauma in accounting for mental disorders throughout the life cycle, in identifying the two-trauma mechanism, and in the conceptualization of early traumatic events relating to the development of Borderlines, Schizophrenia, PTSD, Autism, Symbiosis and other disorders—forcing academics to reevaluate our thinking." He added that the research is respectable, adds to the arguments, and is in support of the model.

Bob Cancro, chief of Psychiatry at the New York University Medical Center, reviewed the textbook for the *American Journal of Psychiatry*. In a personal letter he wrote, "One must always separate statistical significance from clinical significance. Having said that, when a statistical significance is replicated on different samples, it strongly suggests an underlying clinical relationship. I believe this has been done in the data."

I approached the five above-mentioned experts because I considered each to be the foremost leader in his field at the time. Yet despite their high endorsements, this work remains relatively unknown.

The continued resistance to these findings, for forty years since their initial discovery, is understandable because they counter heavily funded research in the field and indicate that nearly everyone is searching in the wrong direction for cause. Who is left to welcome such findings?

In 1998, I analyzed thirty-four biological research studies presented at an American Psychiatric Association meeting in an attempt to review a complete cross-section of current biological research. I showed how each biological change more likely is the result of a psychological process and not the cause (See Appendix). Only a few studies were omitted, and this was because of redundancy.

The editor in chief of the *Schizophrenia Bulletin* was impressed with the article, but wrote that no one at NIMH could review it because all were biological scientists and therefore would not endorse a finding that biological change is the result of a psychological process instead of the cause.

Imagine that? *No one in the peer-review process at the National Institute of Mental Health could entertain even the possibility that a psychological problem could have a psychological origin!*

To hold this work back because it presents a view that differs from attempts to prove biological cause is not only unscientific, but it is highly unfair to the vast number of people and their families who suffer as a result of these infirmities, and it is unfair to future generations who need to be protected from them.

This does not mean that the remarkable neurobiological findings are unimportant. They truly are amazing, and they stand alone as testimony to the development of biological research technology. The studies themselves help confirm the shift to earlier developmental brain and the shift away from later developmental brain, but they have not been examined from this perspective. Also, since a chain can be broken at any link, the research might lead to a means of interrupting some of the pathways, and the research instruments themselves might be utilized to measure the recovery process and even used as neurofeedback instruments to retrain the brain.

The more we know about the complete process, the easier it is to treat. But to omit a factor that has a one-to-one correlation with the later development of the disorder is a shameful thing for those in the scientific community who might have ignored it for selfish reasons.

To say "might have" is as kind and gentle as I can be, under the circumstances. No reasonable person can deny that an awesome amount of money is funneled into the health care community, and where there are "riches" temptation thrives. As bright and devoted as some professionals are, the human factor is an inescapable reality.

It has been my repeated finding that *original goals of institutions ultimately are replaced to meet the needs of persons running them.* This is in keeping with the statement that no man can serve two masters. Regardless of one's personal beliefs, this appears to hold true.

Drug companies search for cause as long as it relates to something they can sell; NIMH searches for cause as long as it is biological (they receive 1.3 billion each year from Congress, much of which is for biological research); and the National Alliance for Mental Illness (NAMI)—hurting from unfair blame—searches for cause as long as God did it because if it is not an act of God, it might cause parents to feel worse. (My heart goes out to families because they really suffer.)

So the Big Three, searching for cause, have eliminated cause from the search!

I do not mean to detract from the spectacular, space-age research, or the sincerity and integrity of the men and women doing the studies. What I am saying is that in terms of cause, they are looking in the wrong direction.

For many years, I was puzzled how could it be that nearly the entire field appears to be off course and looking in the wrong direction for cause. Then I read that this same phenomenon has existed for millennia. Isaiah wrote, thousands of years ago, "I am the Lord that turns wise men backward and makes their knowledge Foolish."

Whatever the cause, this appears to be the case with modern-day psychiatry. Once the billions of dollars of research findings and mountains of peer-reviewed articles are placed in proper perspective, prevention will be a reachable goal—because the concepts presented here, when finally recognized, are not difficult to understand.

This big discovery is: BABIES NEED MOTHERS! Who shouldn't know that? *Babies are very susceptible to separation traumas and must be protected from them.*

If there is no separation trauma during infancy, there can be no delayed posttraumatic stress disorder from infancy, therefore no shift to earlier brain, no increase in dopamine, no cognitive deficits, no brain atrophy, etc.

The advent of the working mother in America is no monetary gain to family or to nation. It results in many families spending their life savings on mental health care for their children; and the cost to the US government, in terms of treatment and loss of productivity, is approximately 85 billions each year *for schizophrenia alone!*

<u>Prevention</u>

If the arguments prevail, regarding the delayed posttraumatic stress disorder model, then we have identified, for the first time, a means of preventing schizophrenia and other serious disorders at three distinct levels.

We can prevent or modify the original trauma; we can prevent or modify the second trauma in the vulnerable adolescent and thereby prevent an initial onset of psychosis or depression; and with proper understanding, we can prevent a recurrence in those who already have a disorder.

<u>Summary of Similarities between Delayed Posttraumatic Stress Disorder from Infancy and from Adult Life</u>

1. The original symptom-defining trauma is an overwhelming event.
2. The initial symptom-precipitating trauma matches or resembles the original symptom-defining trauma in some way.
3. The symptom-precipitating trauma triggers a survival mechanism that applies to all life-threatening traumas, for all species, and enhances survival more often than not.

4. The survival mechanism can be maladaptive, in both war trauma and in schizophrenia.
5. Both return *partially* to the entire earlier gestalt, i.e., the earlier mind/brain/reality/feelings/behavior/chemistry/physiology/body movements and neuroanatomic sites in the brain that were active and developing at the precise time of the original trauma.
6. The negative symptoms are the same for both.
7. The positive symptoms are the same
8. The precursors are the same.
9. The defensive wall is the same.
10. Precursors and negative symptoms in both are attempts to suppress/repress original trauma.
11. The one-directional correlation is the same. The war didn't start because twenty years later someone had a flashback, and the infant trauma did not occur because twenty years later someone developed schizophrenia, or because twenty years later someone developed neurobiological change.
12. The age of the schizophrenic when the original symptom-defining trauma occurred can be determined clinically, and the age of the combat veteran at the time of the trauma can be determined clinically too because the symptoms relate to traumas of war.

Confirmation of Age-of-origin of Schizophrenia

1. Two large-scale research studies confirmed a correlation between a separation trauma in the first two years of life and the later development of schizophrenia: Sarnoff Mednick surveyed the 6,000 in the Finnish database to test this theory, and Preben Bo Mortensen supplied the data for the 2,669 in the Danish cohort on schizophrenia. This was significant beyond one chance in a million.
2. Four smaller studies confirmed the same and also confirmed the age of origin of psychotic depression and the age of origin of nonpsychotic depression—all beyond the .001 level of statistical significance. And these significant surveys showed that the traumas in the first two years of life, which correlate with the later development of schizophrenia and psychotic depression, are the same traumas that in the next year of life correlate with the later development of nonpsychotic depression.
3. The neurobiological change in schizophrenia is what we should expect to find with a shift of brain activity to earlier developmental

structures and away from later developmental ones. One change can cause a whole series of changes, just as one stone can cause a landslide. But without the return of brain activity to the earlier developmental brain structures that were active at the time of the original trauma, the entire process is unlikely to occur.

4. The partial shift to age-of-origin specific reality, behavior, body movements, and feelings—which match those of an infant at the age traumatized—is perhaps the most convincing of all.

Section II

Autobiographical Sketch

Inward Journey

Gifted Persons Encountered Along the Way

The Cornerstone the Builders Rejected

Chapter 5

Background: Autobiographical Sketch

Born February 13, 1936, in Flint Michigan. Doctors told Mother she had to have an abortion because no one could have a second cesarean operation. "Absolutely not!" was her reply. Thus life began with Mother making medical history.

My mother, Helen McKenzie, was very ambitious. Born in New York City to immigrants from Budapest, she was raised on a farm in Illinois, lived in London for a while, and then studied violin at the University of Chicago. Next to her kindness and generosity was her unique boldness.

I have one sibling, my brother Albert, who is ten and a half months older. He is a true genius with an IQ of 170 and a photographic memory. Since we were toddlers, Mother told everyone, "My boys are going to be doctors!" My thoughts for the future ranged from violinist to forest ranger to mathematician and nuclear physicist, but ultimately I chose medicine. My brother preceded me in medicine and became a dermatologist.

My father, Hughie McKenzie, was a quiet man who first worked as a lumberjack in the north woods of Michigan, then a taxi driver; and then during the war years, he worked in the defense plant. Mother always raved how brilliant he was. He had unique intuitive abilities and was very kind. After his death, Mother saw him in a vision, helping children cross over to the other side. She said he always loved children very much.

Perhaps my openness to the spiritual realm was a result of my parents' influence. They both maintained absolute integrity in all matters and were kind, charitable, and compassionate people. Once, at age ten, I went with Mother to a church, and the preacher asked all those who . . . (and I didn't understand what it was he said), but he wanted them to stand. I now realize that it must have been some kind of an altar call. Without hesitation, I stood, as did a few others in the congregation. I felt no embarrassment whatsoever. It was an automatic response and seemed quite natural. What I remember the most was my mother's total surprise and how she told others about it afterward. That might have been a more important moment in my life than I ever realized.

For many years, Father had a greater influence on me than Mother. I listened to him tell stories of his youth, and because of this, I became interested in the great outdoors. He told stories of his grandfather, known as the bear man because he had trapped 117 bears and he provided venison to the lumber camps for a penny a pound. Father and I took many hunting and fishing trips together, which furthered my interest in the outdoors.

Childhood Idols

During my teenage years, I had three idols: the first was Albert Schweitzer, the humanitarian, missionary, and medical doctor who dedicated the first thirty-five years of his life to study and the remainder to serving as a physician and missionary in Africa. The second was Albert Einstein, whom I admired for his great discoveries, but most of all, for his scientific integrity. He truly had no attachment to any finding. He sought only truth. The third was Roald Amundsen, the Arctic explorer who challenged the harshest of all conditions to travel the road never traveled and ultimately was the first to arrive at the *South* Pole.

Exploring the Unknown

I always enjoyed exploring the unknown As a young child I wandered alone through the woods and the streams of Michigan and rarely followed a beaten path. I preferred to travel where others had not been. This pattern of search and discovery continued throughout life and eventually permeated my exploration of the mind.

Prior to medical school, I studied for one year at the University of Vienna and the Allgemeines Krankenhaus. I also used the opportunity to study violin with the department chair at the Academy for Music. From there, I took many journeys, but avoided guided tours and tourists. I preferred to travel with the natives and to explore on my own. I hitchhiked across Europe and back, venturing as far north as Norway and Sweden. Another time, I traveled by motorcycle across the Alps (over solid ice!) and the Pyrenees to Spain and back. Never again by motorcycle. I didn't dare take my eyes off the road in front of me, and I had no one to talk with along the way.

Twice during my time in Vienna, I traveled through Yugoslavia and down into Italy, Greece, and Turkey, going by train and also hitchhiking. From there, I made two trips into Africa and the Middle East, traveling by bus, train, and boat, and in many places hitchhiking alone across parts of the Sahara. I traveled through Lebanon, Syria, Jordan, and a portion of what is now Israel, then through Egypt, down to Sudan, Libya, Tunisia, and back again—all without sleeping in a bed. Later, I returned to Algeria and Morocco and then on to Israel.

I was young and adventuresome, and I was drawn to the road less traveled. In retrospect, I did not want to walk the same path as everyone else in the field of psychiatry either. It wasn't that I disagreed with what others were doing or that I didn't get along with people; it was that I wanted to explore beyond the known—I wanted to formulate my own thoughts, and I did not want my thoughts to be confined to limits and boundaries set by others.

The Continuation of the Journey During and After Formal Training

Formal education was completed at the finest teaching institutions. This included four years in undergraduate school, four years in medical school, a year of internship, three years of adult and two years of child psychiatry residency training, and four years of adult and two years of child psychoanalytic training.

All the training was mainstream, but my thinking was not always that way. I couldn't accept one concept unless it was consistent with others and met the rigors of close, independent scrutiny.

As I came to the end of my psychoanalytic training, I began my exploration inward and noted that Sigmund Freud himself had made the inward journey. After close scrutiny of his work, I could not find fault with his careful observations. I attributed this to his inward journey. Nearly everyone who studies the mind in depth marvels at what Freud was able to do. I was more interested in how he was able to do it. In his paper on listening, he describes going to an even hovering level of attention, and he attributes his great recall to this technique. This is a description of the alpha brain wave frequency level of consciousness, a light level of meditation, which enhances not only memory but also clarity of mind and creative thinking.

His approach to writing fostered even greater creativity. Each morning he wrote for thirty minutes upon awakening. The next morning, he immediately would begin writing from where he left off. This I believe enabled him to tap into a deeper resource for creative writing and for discovery. When we fall asleep, knowing that we will continue writing upon awakening, we literally access all the levels of consciousness during sleep. This allows for profound guidance during the night and awakening with enlightened thoughts and answers. Chapter 19 on programmed dreams provides special techniques for doing this.

The Inward Journey

I had never considered my study of meditation a spiritual journey per se. I just marveled at the answers I received and the things I could do at a meditation level. Directing the mind to receive answers during sleep was even more amazing. Many of my patients, through applying the programmed dream technique, were able to do even more. I marveled at what the human mind could do. This was a natural extension from the study of the unconscious mind. Eventually, as results challenged the limits of the five senses, a new area of exploration emerged.

Dianna

It must have been an angel who put Dianna in my life. My journey through life would not have been the same without her. We met at the University of Michigan in Ann Arbor while she was studying medical technology and I was in medical school. It was love at first sight. She was—and has remained—a beautiful, loving, caring person, with a marvelous sense of humor.

We were married in 1963 after I completed internship. In many ways, we were different, but we complemented one another. She was a city girl and I spent half my life outdoors. She has been the mother our "babies" needed. She has done a wonderful job with our two daughters, Victoria and Christina, and they adore their mom.

Chapter 6

A Guided Journey?

The next three chapters break from strict linear thinking and delve into the more intuitive, a realm of dreams, visions, and spoken words heard during sleep.

The preface of this book noted that many scientific discoveries came through intuition. These include some of the most important scientific discoveries ever made. For the budding scientist, the next three chapters could be critically important.

I can only trace my own personal movement into the intuitive realm, and question in retrospect whether it was a guided journey. I present this with as much precision as time allows, so you can judge for yourself. Perhaps this will cause you to reflect on your own experiences that you have found difficult to explain.

Early in my career I learned to meditate and also learned to seek information during sleep. Dream programming is formulating a question and deciding to have a dream that will tell the answer. I was amazed at each answer but did not explore deeply to determine how it arrived. It is only after looking back over the last forty years that I see a more cumulative significance and wonder at its source.

When my first daughter was born in 1975, I decided to find her name during sleep. Answers usually came in the first night or two, but for three weeks I kept asking for her name before finally receiving the name Victoria. In the mailbox, that morning, was a single item, an advertisement for the MS Victoria! Coincidence? I thought so at first, but after reviewing forty years of such experiences I am more inclined to wonder if somehow her name was withheld pending confirmation in the mail.

When the next child was born I had been thinking about a particular name for her. During sleep I was told to not call her that. Two days later I received the name Christina. I didn't know I was Christian. I had never thought about that.

On two occasions during sound sleep I heard a powerful, authoritative voice. The first time was in 1969, shortly after finishing residency training. I had few patients and lots of time, so I decided to study stock market analysis. Soon I became so engrossed that it could have become my total focus in life. Earlier in my career I had decided to forego playing bridge, chess or golf, because I knew I could become so engaged in any of these activities that I would devote my whole life to them and never do anything else.

When I began spending too much time studying stock market analysis, early one morning during deep sleep I heard the most powerful, authoritative voice I ever had heard. It had two other features: it came at the speed of thought and there was not an extra word. Thus I can only paraphrase what I was told: "If you invest that the market is going to go up, one day it will drop and you will lose everything. If you invest that it is going to drop, one day it will go up and you will lose. If you manage to win, you are only lining your pockets with your father's money. It's OK for you to invest ten percent."

The third statement really blew my mind. Who was telling me that I would be lining my pockets with my father's money? My biological father had passed away many years earlier, and he never had any money. My parents had spent everything to send my brother and me through college. I knew the voice was referring to a "spiritual father," but I didn't know who that was.

The fourth statement was spoken with kindness and compassion. It was as if I were being told: "If this really interests you, it is permissible—but only in moderation."

That particular voice has awakened me only twice in my lifetime. This first time was to warn me not to get sidetracked. Sidetracked from what? Was I on a mission of some sort? All I knew is that I had a strong feeling I should follow what I was told. Was this just a continuation of my own intuitive decisions to avoid bridge, chess, and golf? And was that even *my* intuition?

There were two other features of this voice: both times the statements were given in four parts. It also waited until it was time for me to get up in the morning. I didn't know if this was out of courtesy or whether it was so I would not fall asleep again and forget what I was told.

It is now three decades since hearing it the first time, and one decade since being awakened by it the second time. I am still wondering what it is. The powerful voice was different. I pondered recently as to whether this might have been an archangel, but this is beyond my range of knowledge to even speculate. A biblical scholar friend said Jesus is supposed to have spoken with great power in His voice. Could it have been Him? Maybe, but in the past, during sleep, He simply appeared and transferred thought. In recent years, I have become more aware of spirituality, and that has intensified my questioning and my search for the source of that authoritative voice. There is no way for me to tell, but it's not like a dream.

Even with that first startling message awakening me during sleep, I did not ponder the source any further at that time. I just thought, "Wow. That was amazing."

Perhaps this is all beyond the range of experience and therefore does not exist to the reader. But when you come to the programmed dream section of this book, you can try it for yourself and see what you get. The answers pertaining to cause and cure of medical problems, which are not yet known in medicine, might amaze you, and so might the answers that include other verifiable facts previously unknown to us.

Throughout my experience in the field of psychiatry, certain observations and revelations stood out that were quite remarkable, and I know others must have observed the same things, yet few showed interest in what I thought were remarkable findings.

In the year 2007, I challenged professionals on two internet sites to view my DVD of 12 precise parallels between delayed PTSD from adult life and delayed PTSD from infancy. Out of 40 who accepted the offer, *none* challenged any of the arguments or their derivations. The very observations, *which make schizophrenia and other serious disorders preventable for the first time*, were not challenged; they were ignored!

I cannot be critical. I was the same way when I set aside the many miracles I saw. They just didn't capture my full attention. I was amazed at each one, but never explored deeper as to how the mind was able to do what it did. Instead of searching for the *source* of the information, I always just thought, "Isn't it amazing what persons can do during sleep?" I realize now that anything that does not conform to our belief system is easily dismissed, because it is foreign. In order to maintain the integrity of our thought process, we must dismiss it. It is only while beginning to compile the chapters for this book that I look back over decades of coincidences, synchronicities, visions during the night, programmed dreams, and even promptings to meditate followed by immediate revelations that I begin to question, in retrospect, the "accidental" aspect of all these experiences. I begin to see some order, some direction, and some guiding principles that apply over and over again.

Other Evidence of a Possible Guiding Force

People have to experience this for themselves. It is not possible to recount forty years of such encounters here, but I will note a sampling of them.

There were times when I was prompted to meditate or to do something instantaneously that would not have occurred to me to do. I didn't question why I was to do these things or who was asking or suggesting I do them. Each time, I presumed the promptings were coming from my own mind, but my actions were followed by an immediate and striking response. Looking back, it was as though some presence was letting me know it was there. This was very odd. I didn't know what it meant. Sometimes when it occurred, it gave me insight and understanding; and at other times, it seemed to be only for the purpose of letting me know it was there.

For example, one time I was walking Suzie, my Siberian husky. It was a very clear night, and my mind was not focused on anything in particular. I was just enjoying the walk and not engaged in any specific goal-directed thought. Suddenly I looked up and said, "Give me a sign!" Where did that thought come from? Why should that occur to me? Instantly, the very moment I uttered the words and looked up, two shooting stars shot across my visual field in exact parallel. Astounding! What is the probability of that occurring? How would you explain that? Is there an explanation? Statisticians can calculate the probability of this occurring during a one-second interval over the course of a lifetime and occurring a split second after having the thought, looking up, and saying, "Give me a sign." Especially since I have never even thought to ask for a sign. A sign of what?

I took this to mean there was some other being that wanted me to know of its presence, and that it knew of the cosmic event that was about to occur. Why didn't it just say, "I'm here and this is who I am." Fortifying the impact of that experience were several others.

Another time, I was just sitting on my sofa, thinking about nothing in particular, when suddenly I was prompted to meditate on what is God. I didn't question where that idea came from. I just thought to myself, "This is going to take a *long* time;" but within a minute of closing my eyes, I heard the words "love, energy, the creative force." It was as if the answer was already there, waiting for me to ask. Previously I had learned to trust the answers received that way at a light level of meditation because of their consistent reliability. What had prompted me to ask the question? Not only did the answer seem ready and waiting for me to ask the question, but it rang true and it also fit into my then current scientific mind.

Beyond the Unconscious Mind?

Such occurrences were far too frequent to ignore. Repeatedly over the years, there seemed to be a higher guiding force letting me know of its presence in subtle ways.

We live next to woods and fields, and mice invade the house when cold weather approaches. One year I set traps, and by mid-September no more mice were caught. Then the day before Christmas, I looked at a trap and thought, "Oh, don't let one get caught on Christmas Day." None were, but on the morning of December 26, I was stunned to find a mouse in the trap when none were caught for several months. What caused me to have the thought on December 24?

More recently, just prior to Christmas, I wondered if that could happen again. As soon as I had that thought, it immediately was followed by another, "No, because you might think that *you* caused it to happen." Such thoughts most would not think to analyze. Ordinarily we would dismiss these as soon as they occur. But in trying to decipher the coincidences, synchronicities, dreams, and visions during the night, I began to examine the preconscious and unconscious thoughts more carefully. Was all this just part of the unconscious mind? Perhaps this was beyond the unconscious. Why did the first thought occur in the first person and the reply in the second person? That is, why did the first thought come through as "*I* wonder if . . . ?" and the second as "No, because *you* . . . ." The same occurs sometimes in the dream state, especially when dreams are programmed to receive answers to questions formulated the night before. This you will be able to explore any night on your own.

Early one October, after the leaves had fallen, I started writing about the analysis of the direction of flow of love energy. Then a single rose bloomed in the window directly in front of where I typed. At first I thought that was interesting, but it remained in bloom until mid November!

Such events that occurred repeatedly, and defied odds of being coincidental, caused me to examine *everything*, to determine just how much of what occurs routinely throughout each day might be influenced in the same way. I cannot come up with a percentage probability for each thing we think or do or each encounter we have, but I did begin to examine many experiences and believe we can say that *some* things appear directed from outside—and from there I cannot exclude the possibility that *all* things are directed from outside and *nothing* is accidental.

Freud himself had concluded that nothing is accidental, but to him, this meant that everything was under the influence of the *unconscious* mind. The experience with the two shooting stars traveling in exact parallel—coinciding with the spontaneous uttering of the words and looking up a moment earlier—is strong evidence that this phenomenon goes beyond the control of our unconscious minds; and from there, we do not know how all pervasive this influence might be.

As I continued to write about the love energy, I had two incredible experiences during the night: the first was just someone drifting by and uttering the words, "The aura is the edge of the soul." I didn't see the person or being, but I had the sense that it drifted across in front of my visual field from right to left. These were powerful, meaningful words, and they fit into what I was writing at the time.

When people fall in love, they are described as beaming, glowing, radiant, vibrant, turned on. Holy people, who become even more loving, are shown surrounded by light.

Later in life I began reading scriptures and noted they seemed to reflect some of the same experiences and observations—only this was put in terms of "God is light, God is love, let us love one another for love is of God."

I was most appreciative of the visitor who passed by during the night and uttered those informative words, "The aura is the edge of the soul." Apparently the soul is within, and the more a person loves, the brighter it shines.

Before I finished my writing about love, I had another night vision. This was of some highly evolved being, seated before me in a lotus position, surrounded by light, extending arm's length above and to either side, flowing outward and downward like a fountain. Instantly I knew the vision was showing me the elusive fountain of youth, described throughout the ages. It was the outward flow of love energy. When visions like this occur, there is an immediate awareness of what they represent. Simultaneous with the fountain-of-youth awareness was the realization that as soon as you *want* to live forever, you shut off the flow! Love is energy directed outward. Desire is energy directed back to the self. You can want to teach forever, or you can want to serve forever; but as soon as you want to *live* forever, this is *desire*, which is energy moving in the opposite direction.

Two other events make me wonder about protection afforded by that guiding force, and whether our thoughts participate in some way with outcome. These are described under the next two subheadings:

Angels During the Night

There were instances in the lives of my brother and myself when persons tried to harm us, and something unpleasant happened to them. I have often wondered if that was pure coincidence or whether it related to Mother's fervent prayers for our protection.

This whole notion about "coincidental" occurrences is something I've given a lot of thought to. Take for example the time that a political figure was trying to cause me harm. It was totally unjust on his part, and when I learned of it, I experienced a flash of intense anger. Instantly a tingle went up my spine and simultaneously, I somehow knew this scoundrel would find himself in a mess of trouble.

Some time afterward, while asleep, a very strange thing happened. There appeared what I can only describe as a band of angelic beings. Was this a dream? Or was it something supernatural? They did not have wings, but they moved very swiftly. The moment they appeared they simply announced, "We are leaving now." Instantly I blurted out, "Wait! Don't go." Their equally spontaneous reply was, "No. We have finished our work here and are off to another world."

Without hesitation, I fired one question at them, "What religion are you?" I have no idea where that thought came from. My question to the angels was like asking God what religion he was. Their immediate reply was, "None, because religions become fixed doctrines in one direction that have to be broken and then fixed doctrines in another direction that have to be broken."

This entire exchange lasted only about five seconds. I cannot think that fast, nor can I respond so quickly. I was in a deep level of sleep, but totally aware from the moment they arrived, and I had a far greater clarity of mind than during my usual wide-awake state of consciousness. I had analyzed tens of thousands of dreams in my practice, and this was not like a dream.

During this rapid-fire exchange, I was impressed with the element of total love revealed by the fact that the very moment they finished one task, they were off to another. I also puzzled over what they meant by "off to another world" but still do not know.

In the moments after the night vision, I connected the earlier tingle up the spine with the subsequent visit and realized they must have been with me quite some time. This explains why they greeted me by saying goodbye. I also related the experience to the problem with the political figure. All these thoughts came within a minute or two of the night vision. I was stunned by the speed of discourse and realized I myself never would have thought to ask what religion they were.

Between the tingle and the visit, the politician fell off his roof, injured his back, his wife kicked him out of the house, and he was indicted for fraud. I had a strong feeling that judgment was not yet complete, and I actually began to feel sorry for him.

Anger and Forgiveness

One other time, it was an attorney who tried to cheat me, and I was terribly upset by his betrayal. With much anger in my heart, I found myself in the backyard chopping wood and could hardly refrain from picturing his neck on the chopping block. Almost instantly, I was overcome by a realization that I must not engage in such horrific fantasy. Giving up that horror, I created the idea that instead this ruthless attorney should be "blessed" with a case of vomiting and diarrhea.

That night I dreamed about being in a boat and seeing heads floating by. That convinced me I should never wish harm to another human being. The next day I called the lawyer's office. His secretary answered and said, "Oh, he's out with the flu."

Many years later, in a dream, I learned of a power that works through us, but is blocked when we are quick to anger or do not have total forgiveness. This was in answer to a question I had meditated on the night before to learn why I was not developing faster spiritually. I am always quick to fight for justice, and when I see injustice, I can be quick to anger—especially when helpless, innocent people or little children are being harmed. But the dream told me that it is only when we have total forgiveness, are slow to anger, have more control over angry thoughts, and truly mean "Thy will be done" that we are entrusted with greater power. This matched what I learned in the Far East, that a wish made in pure love instantly is granted. The power is there when we achieve total love and when anger and forgiveness are mastered.

Resuming the Journey

My first night vision occurred nearly four decades ago. At three in the morning, I awakened and made the observation that while I was alert, my body was still asleep. What a great time to meditate! Instead of struggling to get to a deep level, I was coming up from a deeper level where I already had been. So I sat up and meditated for a half hour before falling back to sleep. Shortly after falling asleep again, I had my first visitor during the night: His features were slightly more rounded—not fat, but rounded. He held up his right hand in a friendly gesture, smiled, and said, "Hello." Telepathically I knew he said hello, but it was in a foreign language I never heard before, so I repeated the word after him with a question mark. Again he smiled and uttered the same word, and again I repeated it with the same question mark. Once more he repeated the word, smiled, and said, "Do you have to talk so much?"

What a truly cosmic joke and marvelous, dry sense of humor! Only one word had transpired.

Why did that night vision appear? It certainly was a friendly visit. Was it for a purpose? Why did I awaken at three that particular morning? I took it to mean that the entire event might have occurred for the purpose of letting me know that awakening and meditating at 3:00 a.m. was something I should do.

Another time, there was an emergency situation with our younger daughter. She was fourteen, I had just let her older sister go to New York to evaluate colleges there, and our fourteen-year-old thought she should be allowed to do the same. Suddenly one morning, we found she was missing, along with a small suitcase and a duffel bag. We immediately notified the police, and for two weeks, we searched, calling all her friends and asking every psychic I had ever met. One dear friend who had such gifts said, "New York. She's in danger. It is important you find her right away." I called Ronald Hearne in London, a man gifted in the discernment of spirits. He assured me he did not sense that any harm had come to her. Then I called Isabel, the eldest daughter of Jose Silva, who was trained from early childhood to find answers at a meditation level. Immediately, she described my daughter and my daughter's two closest friends as well as I could if they were standing in front of me. Then she said, "She's in a deli on Fifth Avenue in New York City."

I learned to pray as a result of her disappearance, and pray I did. For a while, we thought we had lost her and that she was gone and never would come back again. It was a dreadful feeling. I programmed for a dream to solve this problem, and during the night, I began having a dream about a truck backing into and damaging a garage that was set on pillars and had skylights. I was angered at someone doing that, but the owner of the garage appeared and was remarkably calm about it, taking it very much in stride and noting that it can be repaired. The sense he conveyed of this not being a big issue was remarkable. *It was as though he saw things from a much larger perspective.* Next he was sitting in a lotus position, and there were twelve or fifteen of us sitting in a semicircle in front of him. He gave us seashells, which we inspected and passed around. Then he handed out little transformers, about the size of the seashells, and we did the same. As I was inspecting one of the transformers, he said to me, "We have *lots* of little transformers . . ." Immediately I knew he was some kind of higher being, that the "lots of little transformers" referred to my being transformed into a man of prayer since my daughter's disappearance, and I knew my daughter was safe because no higher being would joke about such a serious matter if harm had come to her. The building that had been damaged was similar to her room that was held above a porch on four pillars on the southeast side of our house, and it had skylights.

Then my brother asked a prophetic priest in California about her, and his reply was, "Ah, my sheep will hear my voice and they will come to me . . . . She is on her way home."

Indeed she arrived home the very next day. Isabel was right. They all were right. She had stayed for two weeks above a deli on Fifth Avenue in New York City with a family she had met there.

Another thing I noticed over the years is that I always seemed to meet the right people just at the right time to move ahead with what I had to do. If I attended a national psychiatric meeting and wanted to meet three or four leaders in the field, invariably I found them without searching for them. This occurred repeatedly. Was this just coincidence? I don't have the answer.

I was particularly blessed with the person I was given to guide me through hazardous pitfalls of the world of psychiatry that I had entered. Dr. O. Spurgeon English—a legend in psychiatry, a diplomat of diplomats, perhaps one of the greatest geniuses the field ever has known—was my training analyst and later became friend and personal mentor for thirty years. He reviewed all my findings and everything I wrote, adding pearls of wisdom along the way. Instead of discouraging new ideas, he encouraged every one of them, but added his own note of caution. "People want something new and different, but not too new and not too different."

Was Everything Guided from the Very Beginning?

Perhaps even the way things are remembered could be a function of a higher guiding influence. Certain minute details, over the many years of study, have stood out as clear as a vision, never to be forgotten. These minute details, while not emphasized as being important, eventually came together to provide the basis and the structure for many of the findings regarding serious mental and emotional disorders. For example, during my externship in 1960, I spent time at a small psychiatric hospital near Ann Arbor, Michigan; and one old psychiatrist there commented that when persons have breakdowns, these invariably are precipitated by strife in marriage.

Then in 1966, one little comment by Dr. Margaret Mahler stood out. She said that the origin of *childhood* schizophrenia is in the first eighteen months of life.

This tiny bit of information—coupled with the observation by the old psychiatrist in Ann Arbor Michigan, who linked a nervous breakdown with separation from spouse—provided the first clues to the origin and the precipitating cause of serious mental and emotional disorders.

Why did those two particular little details leave such an indelible impression? Surely thousands had heard or read what Mahler had said, and thousands had made the same observation as the old psychiatrist in Ann Arbor, Michigan. These little words and concepts stood out with the clarity of a vision, never to be forgotten, and eventually came together to form the basis of understanding the cause and prevention of mental illness. Why did these things leave such an indelible impression? This too causes me to question whether our paths are guided.

The Mysterious Source of Help: Is it Real or Just Coincidence?

I didn't have any of the answers at the time, and I don't have many of them now. But by coincidence in 1999, as I was pondering these questions, a group of ministers contacted me because they wanted to take their community development program to Washington DC for funding, and they wanted me to head their mental health program. We met at a restaurant and a Rev. Mike was asked to say grace. He spoke like he was talking to someone he knew, like he was speaking to his best friend. It was very personal, and not only did he bless the food and everyone at the table, but everyone in the restaurant as well. I had never heard anything like it before. We became close friends after that, and he always remarked that whenever I spoke, he was hearing scriptures in what I said. I didn't know that. I had not studied scriptures.

On our return trip from Washington DC, one of the ministers asked me if I took Jesus Christ for my Lord and Savior. I replied, "I don't know; I never thought about that, but I will find out tonight. I will program a dream."

In the dream Jesus appeared. I never would have asked him the question that I did, but in the dream I just blurted it out, "So what's wrong with the Buddha?" Jesus didn't say there was anything wrong with the Buddha. He just reminded me of the cross.

My new friend liked that answer. Some of his commentaries I include from time to time to assist those who rely on spiritual help. *Hopefully, this will not be a large obstacle for secular readers.* This material on schizophrenia, depression, and other serious disorders is too important to the reader, and to the world community, to have half the readers blocked from benefiting by it. No one is asking anyone to accept something outside his or her belief system. Nearly everyone has had at least one experience that is hard to explain, and some of us have had many.

As time went on, Rev. Mike introduced me to a ministry and suggested my wife Dianna and I go to one of the crusades. We did so. There were pickets outside the convention center passing out adverse information, but I liked what I saw inside. People were joyful and some were deeply moved by the experience.

I'm not suggesting others follow my next course of action. I'm just relaying what happened, because I want to keep my reporting as accurate as possible.

After the crusade I thought about giving a donation, and considered giving $1,000. I never had donated more than $100, and that was a lot of money to me, so I decided to check the amount at the meditation level. Over the years I had learned to trust and obey that "still small voice," which many people simply call intuition—even though I did not know its source. It took only a minute to reach the meditation level. Immediately I heard $10,000, which put me in great conflict. I called my friend Rev. Mike and told him, adding that Dianna would be very unhappy about that. He just laughed and said: "If God told you to give $10,000, He will tell you how to do it." I approached her very sheepishly and said: "Guess what I got at a meditation level?" Her response was tinged with more than a little sarcasm: "Sure." "Give him your Social Security check!" That was the answer!! I had just turned 65 and was about to receive my first social security check. It was like found money, and by the end of the year it would cover the $10,000.

I always felt good about giving, and I never gave for the purpose of receiving something in return although I was told this would happen. By coincidence, we had been trying to sell our farm in the Pocono Mountains. Land was selling for $1,500 per acre. Suddenly the county decided they wanted it, and we managed to hold out for $5,500 per acre. Coincidence? I don't know. Then before closing, a plea came from the ministry for extra funds for a foreign crusade. I provided a little more. At settlement, the county agreed to drop the county transfer tax, and the real estate agent (a personal friend) refused to accept the larger commission I offered him for the good job he had done. The difference was exactly a hundredfold the amount I had just donated.

Another time, when a crisis was happening in my life and Rev. Mike was helping me with prayer, I was awakened the next morning by my saying out loud: "Thank you Jesus." I don't remember any part of a dream, but all the worry disappeared—as though at some deep level there was an absolute awareness that everything would be OK.

The fourth time I had a dream or vision related to Christianity, it was so remarkable that even a person with no belief system at all would have to say that something unusual was happening. It started one night when I was sitting on my sofa, relaxing, and thinking about the 2.9 million families in America, suffering unnecessarily from schizophrenia. Suddenly a prayer blurted out: "Lord, I am sure I wasn't given this information for my amusement. I need funds: funds for research and funds to bring this work forward." That prayer was so automatic that it startled me. I hadn't even thought about praying.

Two nights later I again was sitting on my sofa when I heard (mentally) a one-word directive: "Meditate." I closed my eyes and within one minute had an incredible vision. Ordinarily I can't even picture a doughnut. Although the vision lasted only a second and was an unusual geometric design, it was so indelibly etched in my mind that I immediately made one out of clay. It was a ring with three sides, but the three sides are one continuous side and the three edges are one continuous edge!

This symbol was the farthest thing from my mind. I never would have thought of that. It is the *Symbol of Infinite Oneness*. Mind, body and spirit are one. We are all one. To the Christian it represents the Holy Trinity. The three are one. "May they all be one, as you are in me and I am in you, may they be one in us." To me it is a holy symbol, given by God, through vision, in answer to prayer.

This symbol is so difficult for persons to visualize, that I have placed diagrams of it on the *last page* of this book. Ordinarily persons study it endlessly, with everyone looking over their shoulder, trying to count the sides. Scarcely anyone is able to recognize that it has only one side and one edge.

Immediately following the vision I realized it was the answer to my request for funds to bring the work forward and to do the research. Therefore 100% of the funds derived will go exclusively for that purpose.

I also take this vision as an endorsement and a confirmation of the validity of the findings reported in this book.

There is one more unusual thing about the *timing* of this work: I had a dream in 2007 about climbing a mountain, and I was only 10 or 12 feet from the top—which represented completion of this book. There was a mudslide coming down but it was not hitting me. In the dream I was supposed to connect the slabs of mud with toothpicks. During the dream I was given the interpretation: The slabs of mud represented my writings coming down from above, and the toothpicks represented biblical truth! Where is this coming from? What I do not recall writing at the top of the page, above where I wrote the dream, were the words "Bombings that surprised everyone." I certainly hope this is not so. It could mean there would be bombings in this country around the time it is released.

The summation of these experiences led me personally to believe there *is* a higher guiding power and that this higher power presents in many ways and many forms, but has certain consistent features. In all instances, I have found the encounters useful, helpful, and informative, revealing information I had not known. They are kind, loving, and compassionate, sometimes giving warnings or revealing the outcome of wrong choices, but always leaving the choice to us. It puts the right people in our path when we need them. It lets us know of its presence in countless subtle ways—usually gently, but sometimes quite forcefully, and it entices us to seek its guidance, but does not impose its will. It allows us to have dominion and make our own choices. If we want help, we must ask, but it is there for the asking!

Each must seek and find truth for oneself. Most of us simply accept whatever beliefs we were exposed to early in life—or we reject them totally because of the way they were forced upon us. Once you begin programming dreams and receiving incredibly accurate information about any problem you encounter or decision you have to make, or learn to tune into that intuitive voice during meditation and consistently receive accurate information, you will begin to trust the answers you receive. Even Sigmund Freud—who regarded religion as the opiate of the masses—said that if he reasoned one answer but intuitively thought another, he followed his intuition. I am only exploring the *source* of that intuition.

For many years, I attributed any unique capacity that I had, for my work in psychiatry, to four factors: (1) the many years of academic training and the outstanding teachers who helped along the way, (2) after training, moving completely away from the group mind of the psychiatric community in order to see something different—because you cannot see a cloud when you are in it; you must first separate from the cloud in order to catch its outline and see beyond, (3) training in meditation and in receiving answers during sleep as a means of creative thinking or receiving higher knowledge, and (4) pure undivided love for patient and family as the single purpose for finding what caused the problem and how to solve it.

Eventually, with coincidences, synchronicities, visions during the night, promptings to meditate, one door closing and two more opening, I began to suspect that much, if not all, was being directed from a higher source, and that source could be more important than the other four factors combined.

In my many years of practice, I observed what I can only describe as a faithful, compassionate supernatural force that always is helpful, caring, giving, providing answers to questions and warnings of dangers through dreams and visions, words during the night, coincidences and synchronicities. This is true love.

I began studying the Old and the New Testaments. What I read matched many of the experiences and revelations I had, particularly about love energy. To me, the astounding accuracy of the prophecies lent great credibility to both covenants. I also realized that contained in the scriptures are formulas for living and for child rearing, for peace, joy, happiness, love, prosperity, health, and longevity. The scriptures also provide formulas for governing nations and for world peace. The wisdom is well concealed, however, so we can accept or reject, depending on the condition of our heart.

Chapter 7

Amazing Spiritual Gifts of Others

Since the early 1970s, I have encountered persons who truly are gifted spiritually. They have been people of all different faiths and nationalities and from different parts of the world. I have been impressed by their wisdom, their knowledge, their love, and their ability to discern truth.

At the same time, I have noted how God-inspired messages can be altered and come to misrepresent the truth they are intended to convey. In Paul's letters to the seven churches, he attests to the frailties of the flesh and shows that even the church can alter God-given messages in a relatively short period of time—but his letters also reveal how a person with divine revelation can discern truth.

The angels in the night vision said it well when they said religions become fixed doctrines in one direction that have to be broken and then fixed doctrines in another direction that have to be broken.

Throughout my journey, I have been deeply moved by those who have demonstrated a powerful communication with the divine.

One such person is Dr. Orest Bedrij. At age twenty-three, he was the youngest member of a team at IBM that was to develop the fastest computer of the day for the Atomic Energy Commission (AEC) and the National Security Agency (NSA). The problem was that if there were billions of calculations to do, the existing computers had to do them one at a time, making the process far too slow. Bedrij knew that total knowledge of the universe exists at every point in the universe (God is everywhere), and therefore he should be able to just *see* the answer.

After two months of collecting information, reaching deep levels of inner peace, going to work every day and interacting with family, he looked up from his desk and saw Boolean equations suspended in midair. He began writing as fast as he could. When he finished, the vision revealed how to calculate all numbers simultaneously, thus solving the problem for AEC and NSA.

Then at age twenty-nine, Bedrij became IBM's technical director at the California Institute of Technology Jet Propulsion Laboratory. He was responsible for hardware and software development for the computer and communication complex that controlled the first soft landing on the moon. They wanted to be on the moon before the Russians, so his team worked feverishly around the clock, four shifts, seven days a week.

To be more effective in his decision-making, Bedrij—with few exceptions—held no meetings and accepted no phone calls until noon each day. He stilled his mind while looking at a large program schedule. In this way he was able to access answers from within for the guidance he needed. In less than a year the center was ready for the moon.

These accomplishments are easily verifiable, but they do not begin to compare with his inward journey and direct communication with the Divine Being within. In one of his scientific papers he writes: "Like Bohr, Wheeler, Einstein, Hawking, Weinberg and many others, we also found ourselves in the land of God, religion and philosophy."

Bedrij affirms that the Divine Being is within *each* one of us, but, to be at one with Him, requires attributes of compassion, purity of heart, kindness and humility. According to Bedrij, it is necessary to move right through the belief *in* Him, to *trusting* in Him, and to the *direct knowledge* and *experience of* the Most High within us. "You don't believe that you breathe, you *know,*" he states.

After twelve years with IBM, Bedrij decided to work on the problem Albert Einstein and other scientists were trying to solve: the unification of existence. He states: "You have to go beyond existence. You have to unify existence with Ultimate Reality, or God in the Highest, of which we are an integral part." For the last thirty years he has been working on this problem. He sees science and religion ultimately coming together, since both seek the unchanging in everything. If it were not unchanging, science and religion would collapse, says Bedrij.

His library has walls filled with volumes pertaining to science, mathematics, Great Books of Western Civilization, philosophy and Holy Scriptures from all major religions. The section on Christianity even has forty-five large volumes from the first 350 years of the church. You can read of his work in *Celebrate Your Divinity: The Nature of God and the Theory of Everything*. Some of his scientific work has been published in English through the National Academy of Sciences in the Ukraine. Scientists, who are searching for the theory of everything, might read his latest publication: *'1': The Foundation and Mathematization of Physics*.

While my journey ultimately has led me to Christ, I was given an opportunity to get to know a true holy man who is the most Christlike person I ever have met. We must be careful not to misjudge all the great saints in other parts of the world. Swami Chidananda remains in continuous love, service, and devotion throughout each day. He is in constant prayer and expression of devotional love and has achieved a God-consciousness that few ever attain.

We hear many warnings about idol worship, and I personally believe these warnings are true. Swami Chidananda speaks of "many names and many forms, but one God" whom he has come to know on a very personal basis. Swami Chidananda is a holy person. His Christmas sermon contains the sweetest, most loving, and most touching writings on Jesus I have seen.

Swami Chidananda is a great teacher and responds to thoughts as soon as you have them. He is revered by his disciples and rightfully so. His voice alone heals. I had a dozen of my most depressed patients close their eyes and listen to a recording of him. They were not able to remain depressed. After reading a pharmaceutical company's boast of improving a depression rating in 61 percent of persons taking their medication for *two months* (as opposed to only 51 percent with placebo), I conducted an Internet survey before and after listening to one of Swami Chidananda's recordings, with eyes closed. Among those responding, 81 percent reported feeling better—*and in only twenty minutes*!

The only other voice I have heard that encompasses as much love, peace, and serenity is that of Pope John Paul II in his new millennium recording. I would like to test that too in similar fashion. I am sure it will achieve the same results. The voice is a reflection of true holiness.

Swami Chidananda also writes that it is a well-known fact that each person is fully responsible for all of his actions. Responsibility rests directly on that person's shoulders. Then he adds, "But I take no action. Therefore I have absolutely no responsibility." This is startling at first because many regard him as the spiritual leader of India. What he means, of course, is that the actions are not his. They come as a result of direction from above and his total obedience to that direction.

My last visit with him was on their highest holy day in March 2000. The Sivananda Ashram in Rishikesh, India, was crowded with thousands of devotees, some of whom had walked for days to come to the celebration. It was also a very special day because he was retiring as president of the Divine Life Society. When we were parting after a very lengthy visit, he noted that the people had been waiting to honor him for nearly three hours.

While we are privileged to know Jesus, it is written, "Seek and ye shall find"—and there were persons all over this earth for many thousands of years who did that very thing.

My younger daughter told about taking a trip out West with two friends in a VW Bus. Suddenly the motor sounded like it was going to fail and they would be stranded. Then since they were in American Indian territory, she joked, "Let's pray to the Great Spirit." So they did, and when they pulled into a rest stop, an American Indian chief approached their VW Bus and said their engine didn't sound right. He worked on it for a couple of hours and fixed it. They thanked him, and as they drove off, he said to them, "Keep praying to the Great Spirit."

Such events as these often are the beginning of a spiritual journey. Was this the Holy Spirit (?) saying, "I'm here, I'm here?" There probably is no limit to the ways in which we are reached. But discernment is critical because evil can pose as good. Too often we see the spec in the other person's eye, however, and miss the log in our own. Many condemn anything that does not fit exactly within very limited boundaries of their own experiences.

There are many ways in which the Spirit communicates with us and with different peoples in different parts of the world.

Christians are waiting for the Second Coming of Jesus, and they believe he will destroy false doctrines. According to Abdullah Yusuf Ali, Muslims too are awaiting the Second Coming of Jesus in the last days, and believe that he will destroy the false doctrines that pass under his name. Jews also are awaiting the Messiah, and a small but growing number believe it might be Jesus. There are widely divergent views as to who how where when and what, but most of the world professes to believe He is coming. When you read chapter 19 you will be able to find clarification for yourself through the programmed dream technique. It is easy. I have never known a person to get a wrong answer. Just decide, "I will have a dream about the Messiah, and the dream will tell me who he is and will tell the truth about him." Don't be surprised if you get a personal visit!

Another amazing saint I have come to know and love is Pastor Patti Damus Perior who, for nine and a half years, did the California wheelchair ministry for Kathryn Kuhlman. When Patti was born, the doctor told her mother, "You won't have her long. She has a hole in her heart and babies with this only live eighteen months." Indeed at eighteen months, Patti had a grand mal seizure. Her mother carried her into town, and as she was walking over a bridge, the Lord instructed her to go under the bridge and baptize her in the river below. She obeyed and dedicated Patti's life to Jesus.

At age nine, Jesus appeared at the foot of her bed and said to her that in the morning she could tell her mother that He had healed her. Patti always had been ashen gray and never could do anything physical. The next morning, her cheeks were pink and she was completely healed. Decades later, as Patti was telling this story, her brother began crying. She asked what the matter was. He revealed that he had walked past her bedroom that night, and he saw Jesus standing there too!

Patti leads the Life in the Spirit Ministry in Porter Ranch, California, where miracles are the norm. Many are healed and come to know the Lord.

I was privileged to travel throughout Israel with Patti and her husband, Tim Perior, in November 2005. We visited various shrines and holy places. While at the Garden Tomb, Patti began telling me about her son running up to her one day, shouting, "Mommy, look at my lizard, I always wanted a lizard." The lizard was dead and rigor mortis had set in. The child next ran into the kitchen to show it to the maid who said, "Get that thing out of here. It's dead, it's rotting, and it stinks." The child ran back to Patti and said, "Mommy, will you pray for it for me?" Patti, who is in continuous dialogue with the Lord throughout each day, did not want to touch it—but she heard the Lord say, "Hold it by the throat." She obeyed. It came fully back to life, the maid screamed and ran out, and Patti heard the Lord say, "I wanted to show you the resurrection power." The maid had been brought in for a witness.

Then Patti said to me, "I don't know why I'm telling you this." I am sure it was because we were at the resurrection site. She is precious beyond words. Total love, compassion, humility, and as sweet as can be. Only Jesus could be sweeter. From the very first moment we met, we were the best of friends. I refer to her affectionately as my shy, timid giant.

Another amazing holy man I met long ago was Swami Kripalvananda, in Ahmadabad, India. Many considered him the most highly evolved Kundalini Yogi in India at the time. In December 1973, I received a letter from him saying that I could visit the next week. I was excited for the opportunity to meet with him.

The night I received his letter, I went to bed with the thought of asking him how to become total love toward all people all the time because I reasoned if we could take the most intense experience of love we ever had, multiply it a thousandfold, and experience it toward all people all the time, what an incredible state of bliss that would be! I further reasoned that there should be nothing to prevent this because love comes from within. This wish was followed by a strange experience during sleep in which I actually felt like I was becoming that love energy.

When I met with the swami the next week and asked how to become total love toward all people all the time, I thought he never would stop laughing. When finally he regained his composure, he wrote on slate with chalk—because he had not spoken for thirty years—and a disciple translated, "When you want to hit a target with an arrow, you aim only at the bull's eye!" This made perfect sense. We reach out with a love-need combination, and because our needs can be hurt, we do not reach to our full capacity. But if we direct our love toward God, there is no rejection, and therefore we can reach more fully. Furthermore, we begin to emulate Him to whom we reach.

Thirty years later I found this "aiming at the bull's eye" stated in Scripture: "So I run straight toward the goal in order to win the prize . . . ."

Then I asked the swami what I should do next, thinking that he would give me a meditation technique that would bring me to enlightenment. Again he laughed, then wrote on slate with chalk, and the disciple translated, "Just keep doing exactly what you are doing." It is thirty-four years later and finally I am beginning to suspect what he told me back then might be true—that my path has been guided from the very beginning.

This truly was a man of great wisdom. His answers were to love God first and to stay on the path I was following. Where did he get his information?

Another most remarkable person I have come to know is Dr. John Diamond, and his talented and precious wife Susan. Dr. Diamond earned his MD degree in Australia and then worked two years in a state mental hospital, nearly 50 years ago. He loved his 200 patients very much, and even remembers almost every one by name. When he returned many years later he found the hospital torn down. He looked for his patients but could not find them. He was terribly saddened and longed for them.

Why did he love them so much? He had taken photographs of many patients but not because he wanted their pictures. He wanted to look deeply into their eyes, and the camera was just a prop so they would not feel uncomfortable. What did he see that caused him to love them so much? Was it the soul of the innocent child who unknowingly was hurt? He too recognizes the early mother-infant relationship as most crucial for human development.

It is easy to have great compassion and love for a mental patient when the infant, toddler or young child is revealed in them. I feel great compassion, for example, for Casey Anthony, who has been portrayed as an extreme villain, month after month on national television, for the better part of a year. I see a child, less than two years old. This should be apparent by the stories she tells. Others feel compassion too, but cannot explain why. As she comes out of the earlier mind, the adult mind tries to reconcile what might have happened. This is a very sad thing. The hatred of a nation is pointed at her for possibly killing Caylee, her young daughter--but they do not understand. Casey could be anyone's child.

I believe Dr. Diamond saw the precious young toddler or infant in his 200 state mental hospital patients and in so many since. His response to them is a natural response anyone might have to a hurt young child. You want to pick them up, hold them and comfort them.

Dr. Diamond is very sensitive and works with life energy, which he describes as the healing power within each individual. He appreciates and encourages all expressions of the spirit. He is a pioneer in Applied Kinesiology, and in 1976 began using acupuncture meridians in psychotherapy, ushering in the power therapies. He utilizes various art forms in his treatment, and his artwork is exhibited worldwide. His haiku drawings, made during meditation with one single breath, are extraordinary, and transfer a feeling of peace and tranquility to the viewer.

Another spiritual friend I have come to know is Dr. LaDonna Taylor. Our first encounter was at a crusade. She played the violin, and it was the most anointed violin playing I had heard, but the violin she played was not a concert instrument. Two days later, I began having the thought, "Loan her your violin." At first I wondered where that ridiculous thought came from. I wouldn't even let my adult children play that violin. But the thought persisted until I realized its source, at which point I called and told her she could borrow one of my violins.

She told me she had bought a Gabrielli violin and later found it was a fake. Then someone gave her a Peresson violin, which prompted her to give away her own concert violin—but six months later, that person said to her, "I'm taking it back. You don't deserve it." She was crushed and cried for days.

I happen to have two concert violins. Imagine her surprise when I offered a choice of a 1762 Gabrielli violin, perhaps the finest in existence, or one of the best Peressons ever made! Was this a coincidence? Perhaps. But a Gabrielli is rare and there are not that many Peressons. The probability of having both is quite remote.

If we were to try to calculate probabilities, fewer than one in 100 million might have a Gabrielli, and fewer than one in 10 million would have a Peresson. To have both is even more remote, and for her to have previous hurtful experiences with the same two violins is so remote that it is more reasonable to presume divine intervention rather than coincidence.

Dr. LaDonna has a violin ministry, performing every week at churches around the world, and she reports many miracle healings during her services. A number of them are verifiable. I saw one of them myself. Her music brings emotional, physical, and spiritual healing to many. She has just been nominated for the Dove Award and Record Album of the year. Hopefully she will win.

Last year, I met two more very special persons. Both are healers and had their initial experience by age five. One is a retired physician, Dr. Bob (MD/PhD), who reports that he had his first experience in 1947, at age four, when a radio evangelist said, "If you are sick, just place your hands on the radio and receive your healing." He was suffering from rheumatic fever; so he placed his hands on the radio, fell out in the spirit, began speaking in tongues, and was totally healed. He has continued to speak in tongues every night since, and many miracles occur through his ministry. The other friend is an eighty-four-year-old woman, Martha Moore Stevens. She had her first experience at age five when she was in excruciating pain, all alone, and was dying. Her parents never went to church; but when she visited her grandparents, her grandfather, a Baptist minister, would always point to a picture of Jesus and say, "If you ever need help, just call on Jesus." So she said, "Jesus, if you are real, come and help me." She reports that He came, held her hand, and said, "What would you like me to do?" She asked if he could heal her, and immediately he did. Then she asked, "Gee, can I do that too?" He told her she could, she asked how, and he said, "Just follow the path of love."

Both of these delightful people are reported to have unique healing abilities, and many of their healings are medically documented. Dr. Bob and his wife Judy devote their lives to helping people. Martha did her healing by telephone and never charged. Sadly, she passed away recently. She earned her living by making healing quilts.

These are just a few of the saintly persons who have crossed my path and have added inspiration and meaning to my life. I have included them because my own experiences are more limited, and I wanted to give you a wider range of expressions of the spirit within. There are many more, and this journey becomes more interesting and rewarding all the time.

Chapter 8

The Cornerstone that the Builders Rejected

The cornerstone was prophesized in Isaiah 28:16: "Behold, I lay in Zion for a foundation a stone, a tried stone, a precious cornerstone." David declared it in Psalm 118:22-23, "The stone which the builders refused is become the head stone of the corner. This is the Lord's doing; it is marvelous in our eyes." This is repeated in Matthew 21:42.

Isaiah was condemned and rejected for his prophesies and David lamented that everyone troubled him and rose up against him saying there is no help for him in God (Psalm 3:1-3). Jesus was totally condemned and rejected, as the light of the world, for his beliefs. He later became the cornerstone and the head of His church.

I have found, in similar manner, that anyone who tries to bring light or revelation knowledge into any aspect of life can be condemned and rejected.

I am not a prophet and I do not put myself in that category, but I do believe I bring a measure of truth to the field of psychiatry.

To say I was rejected puts it mildly. Virtually everywhere I have gone, since entering psychiatric residency training in 1963, I was flatly rejected—not for doing anything wrong, but for having new ideas or not rubber-stamping the old.

During my first year of training at the Menninger School of Psychiatry in Topeka, Kansas, my supervisor thought I was not suited for the task. He himself had been forced to leave Menningers but returned to work there after he received training elsewhere. Another supervisor thought I would never understand psychodynamics. He didn't realize that I was not rejecting psychoanalytic principles; instead I was carefully reviewing them for accuracy, making sure that each was valid. This differs from accepting a premise because it is peer-reviewed or because some person, important in the eyes of man, wrote it.

Before my departure, Dr. Karl Menninger called me into his office and told me, "I can't understand it. You are just the way I was." He wished me well and gave me a book he had written on hope.

One door shut, two others opened.

In spite of the rejection at Menningers, in Philadelphia I was accepted directly into the Psychoanalytic Institute; and Dr. O. Spurgeon English—one of the most respected psychoanalysts of the twentieth century—agreed to be my training analyst.

It would have taken several more years to be accepted into psychoanalytic training in Topeka. The move was a huge career enhancement.

During my second and third years of psychiatry residency training at the Philadelphia Psychiatric Center, my work was harshly criticized, and there were efforts to terminate me from that program. I just didn't fit into anyone's mold. I had to see and test things for myself, and would not compromise my findings. It was a struggle just to complete the training there.

After completing the four didactic years of adult and the two years of child psychoanalytic training, the psychoanalytic institute decided I was not suited for that kind of work. I had begun to explore psychodynamics of groups and of nations, and this led to exploring and writing about the psychodynamics of psychoanalytic groups. To question the psychodynamics of psychoanalytic training was not acceptable.

But this too was fortunate because had I stayed for the completion of the required number of supervised psychoanalytic patients, my thoughts might have been limited. I was not critical of the teachings. Nor did I disagree with Freud's careful observations. But there was a danger of becoming so inundated with psychoanalysis that I might just continue to add more and more to Freud's observations when there were other dimensions to explore. We cannot see a cloud when we are in it. We must separate from it in order to catch its outline and see beyond. It was necessary to leave this pursuit.

As I continued to explore new territory, I began to notice telepathic abilities in some psychotic patients and in children. I experimented with my child psychiatry patients and made it part of their play therapy. Some exhibited amazing accuracy well beyond chance. I corresponded with Anna Freud, and she expressed great interest in the findings. We entertained the possibility this is how young children seem to know things they have not been taught. She looked forward to more of the findings, but also noted that in all the psychoanalytic literature, there was only one vague reference to mental telepathy, in a 1935 article, printed first in German, by Dorothy Burlingham.

I was stunned. If the greatest minds, studying the human mind, did not see or dared not report a mental phenomenon reported by 60 to 80 percent of the general population, it was time to get off the academic guided tour bus!

Before long, I had difficulty with the hospital where I was practicing. It was my Philadelphia alma mater. This was still early in my practice, and I spent long hours with my patients, trying to understand the cause of their illnesses and trying to learn what to do to help them. Sometimes I spent all day at the hospital. No one else did that. I would take patients out of the hospital to go places with them. No one else did that either. I began to see what upset my patients in everyday life, what precipitated their initial breakdown, and how this related to their early history. No one else was exploring the same things. I was not part of the herd. My findings were foreign to them. I didn't understand why they couldn't see what I thought were obvious findings and simple concepts, and they couldn't understand why I didn't treat patients the way everyone else did. They couldn't understand why I would take a patient out of the hospital for a pizza and a beer across the street, or why sometimes I would separate a patient from family. They also did not understand my exploration of consciousness itself. This might have troubled them the most. It was beyond their range of experience.

It was fortunate they didn't hear about my taking a patient out of the hospital for an exorcism. Alan Neuman, a Hollywood movie producer, called and asked if I had any patients who were possessed. He wanted to film a live exorcism, which he had asked Fr. Eugene Gallagher to perform. Fr. Gallagher, former chairman of two departments at Georgetown University, is the priest who did one of the exorcisms in the true story behind the movie *The Exorcist*. By coincidence, I had two patients who spoke in another voice—not a regressed schizophrenic voice, but an evil demonic-sounding voice that matched the voice in the movie. I provided the patient.

I learned that if you do something different, people will start to take note and will begin to talk. That's all it takes. From there, the gossip mill just keeps churning out bigger and better stories. A person doesn't have to do anything wrong. All it takes is doing something different. This happened at the hospital where I was practicing. The further from the hospital the rumors were generated, the more incredible they became. Then they reverberated back to center and back out again, ever increasing. Soon the hospital tried to limit my treatment of patients to what other staff members thought was right. I understand their feelings, but it was totally frustrating to try to help my patients with one hand tied behind my back. Eventually I wrote an article that appeared in the American Medical Association newspaper, saying that I felt like Jascha Heifetz playing second fiddle to a bunch of amateurs, all of whom agreed they were correct.

Apparently it was obvious which hospital I was criticizing. This set off a fury. Rumors multiplied exponentially. Even the *Psychiatric Times* was targeted for publishing an article I wrote about the American Psychiatric Association's paper selection process, and their advertisements suddenly were stopped. I learned the impetus for stopping those advertisements came from the same group in Philadelphia. Eventually I could not even visit a patient in a hospital where I never had been, had never met anyone, and no one had evaluated my work.

One of my schizophrenic patients became trapped in the mental health care system. His insurance ran out, and the state took over. I traced him through nine institutions where he was all but killed. If the rumor was that I didn't give medication, then he was given mega doses. If the current rumor was that I gave him medication, then medications were withheld. Everywhere he went, he was told terrible things about me. His life was in great danger, and all progress had stopped.

This was no way to treat a confused, delusional patient. He could not understand what they had against me. I was the only one who had been able to explain his psychosis to him in a way that he immediately understood and knew that he knew. He had made great progress and had seen his way out of his serious mental illness. Their actions were very destructive, and he became confused and more delusional as he was transferred from one institution to another.

Earlier, I thought of writing the book *Hung by the Grapevine*; but when I discovered what they were doing to my patients, I became like a mother bear protecting her cubs and decided to yank that grapevine out of the ground. Was I being tested? Was this my lion or my bear? Whichever it was, the other came later and quite a few more. Indeed, this battle with the hospitals probably was my Goliath.

As matters worsened, about a quarter of a century ago, I filed suit against seventeen psychiatric institutions and directors—including the Commonwealth of Pennsylvania and the nine institutions that harmed that patient. On the way to sign papers, I stopped at a Chinese restaurant, cracked open a fortune cookie, and there was nooooo fortune in it. It was as if to say: "*This* . . . is on you!"

Signing those papers was scary. I was inviting a showdown with nearly all major elements of the psychiatric community. Driving home, I began to experience real fear for the first time. Then a strange thing happened. Although I had been exploring consciousness itself, practicing meditation and programming dreams, I never had any religious training and was not familiar with any hymns except for Christmas carols. Nonetheless, as soon as I felt this survival fear, I broke out in song—complete with words and melody; and it is a hymn that, to my knowledge, never has been written or sung. The words are: "Trust in the Lord and all will be well. Trust in the Lord and all will be well. Trust in the Lord and all will be well, and all will be well, and all will be well, and all will be well, and all will be well."

Was I being helped? Where did that come from? Somehow, after singing this little hymn, the fear totally disappeared. The words "and all will be well" repeated seven times, and the fear was gone. Was this more than just *my* battle?

Oh, the outcome with the hospitals? All seventeen paid. After fourteen of my depositions, most of which lasted all day—where I went with my attorney and they appeared with their dozen or so attorneys—they found nothing that warranted their criticisms, and no patient would speak against me. That was a very long time ago, and in retrospect, I realize there must have been a lot of unseen help.

No one person should have been able to win against an entire community. Was it because of some higher guiding power, looking over the multitudes of families desperate for help, that this work prevailed? Who knows? I didn't even consider that possibility at the time. In retrospect, there are many families around the world who suffer unnecessarily from these illnesses. Mental illness can be prevented and can be treated, and the immense suffering of all family members, which few fully appreciate, must be recognized and stopped. Perhaps it was a higher power that intervened.

Section III

Review of Parameters for Measuring Age of Origin

Other Searches for Cause

Age of Origin of Other Symptoms and Diagnoses

This section reveals various parameters for determining clinically the age of origin of symptoms and diagnostic categories. In contrast to the *Diagnostic and Statistical Manual*—which affixes diagnostic labels to various symptom categories—this system delineates origin in terms of the month when the symptom-defining trauma occurred.

From there the degree of illness is measured by the percentage shift to earlier mind and brain, and how long the person remains ill.

The next chapter explores other searches for cause, and notes that none other identifies cause that appears to relate to all schizophrenia, and without which schizophrenia is unlikely to occur.

Lastly we search the age of origin of specific symptoms and diagnostic categories, and we explore and expand the findings to nearly all other categories of mental and emotional conditions.

Chapter 9

Brief Review Plus Age of Origin of Other Early Parameters

There has been an explosion of knowledge in the mental health field in recent decades, but with each particle racing farther from the core. Each particle then gathers followers, but the followers are not necessarily the scientists. And they might have special interests, which isolate the particles further, and instead of integration, we get fragmentation.

To cloud the picture further, billions of research dollars in recent decades have been spent searching for biological cause while comparatively nothing has been spent searching for psychological origin. In the search for biological cause, not only are there institutional backings and broad-based funding, but there are very impressive-looking and highly sophisticated pieces of equipment such as PET scans and digital and functional MRI. This helps create the false impression that biological research is more scientific, that biological change produces the disorders, and that the study of the mind is but a pseudoscience.

Countering this now is data on the 6,000 in the Finnish database on schizophrenia, the 2,669 in the Danish cohort on schizophrenia, and the hundreds more surveyed by Dr. Lance Wright and myself. These surveys confirm a correlation between a five-day separation trauma during the first two years of life and the later development of schizophrenia.

In order to integrate the fragments of mental health research that seem scattered in all directions, and in order to identify cause, we started with the most dramatic of the mental disorders, namely, schizophrenia, where the symptoms are pronounced and relatively easy to see. Once these are recognized, the more subtle forms of illness can be identified

Then we looked at the simplest of all psychological mechanisms that many already understand, namely, posttraumatic stress disorder from adult life. Most have heard stories about combat veterans who become startled and immediately believe they are back in combat. Even without psychological training, this is easy to understand.

In the case of combat veterans, we noted that posttraumatic stress disorder (PTSD) is a survival mechanism in which the veteran goes onto automatic pilot when a threat occurs, which is similar to the original terrifying war experience.

Then we noted that to the infant, separation from the mother can be as threatening as war trauma to a soldier because to mammalian babies—for as long as mammals have populated the earth—separation from mother has meant death.

Next we looked at *delayed* PTSD and saw how earlier mind and brain could be activated later in life and then reactivated over and over again with little further provocation. We considered how this could alter patterns in the brain, especially if the trauma were from a very early age.

Most who observe the shift to infancy simply regard it as *un*reality instead of *earlier* reality.

When I encountered this for the first time, it was as a small child back in 1941. An eighteen-year-old girl was running nude through the lawn sprinkler in our front yard, squealing with delight. I was puzzled and thought, "What's wrong with her? Grown-ups don't do that." It took a quarter of a century to realize this was perfectly normal behavior, but transposed in time. Had she been eighteen *months* old instead of eighteen years old, no one would have thought anything odd about her behavior.

With the combat veteran, there is a shift to war experience, reality, feelings, and behavior; and there also is a shift to the corresponding physical, biochemical, and physiological response. The same regions of the brain are reactivated, literally the same brain cells, and these still are hardwired to the rest of the body. The heart beats faster, the person breathes harder, pupils dilate, hands and feet perspire, and the adrenals pump adrenaline into the bloodstream. There is a very dramatic remembering and re-experiencing, even at cellular and subcellular levels; and the person literally flashes back in part to the entire earlier gestalt—i.e., the earlier mind/brain/reality/feelings/behavior/chemistry/physiology/body movements and neuroanatomic sites in the brain that were active at the precise time of the original trauma during combat.

With schizophrenia, there is a similar shift to earlier times, and the behavior and reality also match the particular earlier age. This reality and behavior varies according to precise age-of-origin.

Body Movements in Schizophrenia

One recovered schizophrenic girl described looking around the room, during her illness, to see who in the room was controlling the movement of her arms. This can only come from the reality of an age prior to realizing that it is she who moves her arms.

Early arm movements are symmetrical, so a person with schizophrenia who suffered a very early trauma might move arms in unison. If the person is walking with arms extended for balance, you know the trauma occurred when the person was learning to walk. If they walk with normal arm movements, this is either from an age subsequent to learning to walk, or it represents only a partial shift to earlier infant brain. If they are walking with arms straight down to the sides with no arm movements at all, they can be at an age prior to learning to walk, or this symptom can relate to the effects of medication.

When the baby first starts moving its arms about, it has little control and it might hit itself in the face with its fist or scratch its face with its fingernails. One such young man was terrified of hitting himself in the face with his fists or scratching his face with his fingernails. This fear obviously came from trauma at a time prior to gaining control of his arms.

This lad had suffered a traumatic birth with lack of oxygen, causing brain damage, and he was adopted shortly after delivery. Eventually, thirty years ago when shock treatment was in vogue, this modality was applied. After the third treatment, his tongue protruded from his mouth and food dropped out of his mouth onto his lap when he tried to eat. At first, I considered the possibility that he fractured his neck, but then I learned that the treatment team was unable to give him oxygen prior to that third treatment. I then realized the lack of oxygen took him to anoxia at birth, which took him to an age prior to learning to eat solid food, and this accounted for the tongue protruding forward and pushing the food out of his mouth. Prior to learning to eat solid food, the infant sucks by pushing the tongue forward in the mouth. So instead of ordering an X-ray to rule out a fractured neck, I ordered the next treatment and the symptoms disappeared. With the sixth treatment, the symptoms reappeared; and once more, I learned that the treatment team was unable to administer the pretreatment oxygen. Again, with the next treatment it disappeared. This identifies his symptoms as having an origin prior to learning to eat solid food (tongue pushing forward in his mouth) and more specifically relating to birth (anoxia).

The intensity of the fear of scratching or hitting the face, incidentally, was augmented by the severe birth trauma—which had served as an antecedent trauma, making the later trauma more frightening.

Another patient, a young woman, sitting in the hospital cafeteria, was pushing an egg salad hoagie into her mouth as she made short, rapid chewing movements with her jaw. At the same time she was wetting herself. The striking thing was that she experienced the soiling herself while eating to be perfectly normal. She was a multitasking infant who was breast-feeding and wetting her diaper at the same time.

Each bizarre action of the psychotic matches in some way that of the infant at the precise time of the original trauma. Some of the realities, body movements, and behaviors are specific to a particular month or even to a precise moment, while others might apply to an age range-of-origin.

<u>Age of Origin of Other Realities</u>

Reality also depends on age of origin. If there is an infant in a room full of adults, everybody is watching the baby. When a person revisits that reality, the person knows everyone is watching.

How specific in time can this be? To the precise moment when first traumatized. Recall the full-grown man upside down in a fetal position trying to force his head through a toilet bowl? Re-experiencing birth is highly specific. Another person, carrying on a normal conversation, was experiencing pressure and pain around her face, head, neck, and shoulders. I timed her. This was happening every six minutes. We learned that her mother was given general anesthesia during delivery, and I would wager that she was anesthetized when the contractions were six minutes apart. That's how precise this mechanism can be. With delayed posttraumatic stress disorder, the person returns in part to any reality and behavior of the earlier time whether from infancy or adult life.

One recovered schizophrenic woman described hitting her head on the floor and thinking that the floor came up and hit her in the head. This obviously was a very early reality, originating prior to learning to stand, prior to experiencing the law of gravity. It was at an age when perhaps the baby was in a bassinet that tipped over.

A middle-aged woman was convinced that the birds outside her hospital room were robots that were sent to spy on her. In searching for origin, I asked her what age is it that a baby, sitting in a high chair, cannot distinguish between a puppy and a windup toy moving across the floor.

This is the kind of question one must ask when trying to explain origin.

One young man spoke of a fecal man who was all-powerful and who controlled the whole world. As he was coming out of his delusional state, I began first to note that he was experiencing the world differently than he did the previous day and questioned if tomorrow he might experience it differently still. He considered this possibility.

This is a critical time to explore realities, as the person is coming out of a more delusional state. Then I began to describe to him a busy mother who is hassled by having to care for other children and do the housecleaning and grocery shopping and cooking the meals and who is particularly tired of changing smelly diapers. Meanwhile, the mother is the whole world to the baby, but the baby does not seem to be able to do anything to get this busy mother's attention. Then one day he makes a little deposit in the potty. His mother is overjoyed and makes a huge fuss over him, and lets him believe that this is the biggest event in their lives. Certainly, it received by far the greatest positive response ever from her and she is the most important person in the world to him. Suddenly that little deposit becomes the most important thing in his world. It carries magical powers that win him all kinds of praise from his whole world.

The patient was well enough to catch the analogy, yet close enough to the delusional reality to make use of the interpretation. He was still partly in the infant mind, which was important, because the interpretation must be made at the level the patient is experiencing. This is the most critical time for making interpretations to a psychotic individual. The next week he was able to joke about the fecal man, fully realizing its delusional origin.

Not all the age-specific realities observed over the last forty years have been confirmed statistically on a month-to-month basis, but we have confirmed the broad general category of psychosis as correlating with trauma in the first two years of life. Independent, world-class researchers have provided data that verifies this—but they failed to comprehend and appreciate the implication of their own findings. What prevents them from seeing the simple concepts that by now the average reader understands?

On a smaller scale, but highly significant nonetheless, we have confirmed that the identical traumas in the next year of life correlate with the later development of nonpsychotic depression.

More specifically, it has its origin between twenty-four and thirty-four months. To avoid psychosis and depression, you can use babysitters or daycare at thirty-five months. Dr. Benjamin Spock, the pediatrician who spent six years studying psychoanalysis and whose book on child rearing sold 50 million copies, was very attuned to the needs of children. He recommended thirty-six months before starting daycare.

Age of Origin of Early Developmental Brain Reflexes and Learning Opportunities

The powerful mechanism of ontogeny recapitulating phylogeny does not stop suddenly at birth. The infant begins using first the earlier developmental regions of the brain, the brain stem, or the reptilian brain plus the old mammalian brain. The Moro reflex is that of a reptile, for example. Slam your hand on the table and the baby's head rears back and its mouth opens.

Have you ever seen a lizard do that? Or a snake? That is from the reptilian division of the brain. This need not involve the debate regarding evolution versus creation. We utilize all parts of the brain, and our brains include areas that are similar to those of lower species.

There has to be at least some of the old mammalian brain operating at birth—otherwise, there would not be the rooting reflex (if the nipple touches the cheek, the mouth turns toward the nipple and opens). One time, I touched a dying man's cheek to see if he were febrile. Immediately his head turned toward my fingers and his mouth opened. His stress and helplessness had returned him to infancy, the infant mind, and the infant brain. People who are very sick do return to earlier times, to remedies from throughout the life cycle. This is seen in the near-death experience in which one's entire life flashes before one's eyes in an instant. Conceivably, the mind and brain are searching all records for any possible solution.

The sucking reflex clearly comes from the old mammalian portions of the brain. Different areas of brain develop at different ages. Balance, obviously, is developing at the time the infant is learning to walk; and so the cerebellum is developing at that time. Language centers undergo massive development when language development is at its peak, and this results in dramatic increase in size of the left posterior superior temporal gyrus with elongation of the fissure. This can be observed on gross examination or on MRI. And there develops a normal asymmetry of the brain, for speed and efficiency. If both sides of the brain had to be used for everything, this would slow our reaction time because it would require communication back and forth across the corpus callosum (the structure that connects the two halves of the brain).

There are windows of learning opportunity as the infant passes through the earlier developmental regions of brain, and if certain abilities are not accessed at the right time, the person might never develop that particular ability. Instant math—in the first two or three years of life—cannot be learned later. Perfect pitch, as the infant passes through that window of opportunity, also cannot be learned later in life. Language development has its special age. For example, young Berlitz had twelve family members who spoke various languages. Each was asked to speak to him in a different language, and by the time he was four years old, he was fluent in twelve languages.

So the infant is using different regions of the brain that are developing at different times. These developmental areas are age-of-origin specific. This is what accounts for the neurobiological difference between the combat veteran and the person with schizophrenia. When the veteran flashes back to a reality experience that occurred when he was perhaps eighteen years old, that experience is recorded in the adult regions of his brain, in the higher cortical structures. But when the person with schizophrenia flashes back to the experience of eighteen months, he returns to earlier developmental brain structures that were active and developing at that earlier time.

We mentioned that these are the structures that produce more neurotransmitters involved in the schizophrenic process, such as dopamine; and when reactivated, they produce more. We also have the factor of age-specific learning: just as the person can learn to walk and talk and learn instant math and perfect pitch at certain ages, the infant who is overwhelmed might develop a unique *ability to produce* specific neurotransmitters at a certain age and reproduce them when returning to that particular age.

Whether it is because of simple reactivation of earlier developmental brain structures or whether it is a flashback to what the infant learned to produce when traumatized in the first two years of life, the person with schizophrenia does activate the earlier brain structures, and these structures then produce more of the neurotransmitters involved in the disease process.

Cognitive Impairment

The corresponding shift of brain activity away from higher cortical centers results in cognitive impairment as well as brain atrophy. One recovered catatonic patient looked back with humor upon his psychosis and in particular his trying for hours to determine how many one-, two-, and five-cent stamps to put on an envelope that required twelve-cents postage. He had been at an age of origin prior to developing the region of brain used for mathematics. Fortunately, he recovered before he developed a permanent disuse atrophy of the later developmental brain structures.

When a person with schizophrenia shifts to an age prior to language development, the language centers in the left posterior superior temporal gyrus atrophy, proportionately more than in any other area.

In schizophrenia, there also is loss of normal brain asymmetry because persons shift to areas of brain that were active prior to specialization from one side of the brain to the other.

Atrophy in the hippocampus relates to smaller cells, not fewer cells, and this supports the concept of disuse.

So a search for how dopamine causes schizophrenia, or how brain atrophy causes schizophrenia, could go on forever because these changes are the *result* of the disease process and not the cause.

Do you get this so far? It's so incredibly simple: the combat veteran and the person with schizophrenia both suffer from posttraumatic stress disorder, but the veteran flashes back to a trauma in adult life while the person with schizophrenia returns to a trauma during infancy. So the person with schizophrenia is using earlier developmental brain structures, the ones that produce more of the neurotransmitters involved in the disease process. And since there is a relative shift of brain activity away from the higher cortical structures, there develops a disuse atrophy—as would occur in any other part of the body not being used. Incredibly simple!

This is presented in much greater detail in *The Unification Model for Mental Illness* (See Appendix).

Research Evidence of Traumatic Origin

In the early 1980s, Dr. Lance Wright and I tested the infant separation trauma theory; and to do this, we took a complete population of sixty persons with schizophrenia from two halfway houses and compared them with sixty persons who would be considered supernormal (no history of mental illness, had full range of emotion, and lived active productive lives). We studied the two groups for one particular infant separation trauma, namely, the birth of a sibling.

These were hard data categories: either they had a sibling less than nineteen months younger or they didn't, and either they were sick enough to be in a halfway house or they were not.

Among the sixty persons with schizophrenia and the sixty who were supernormal, twenty had a sibling less than nineteen months younger. Like the flip of a coin, if separation had nothing to do with the later development of schizophrenia, there should have been approximately ten from each group. But seventeen were from the group with schizophrenia and only three from the supernormal. This is like flipping a coin twenty times and having it come up heads seventeen.

Then we surveyed the next twenty supernormal individuals we encountered, and only one of them had a sibling less than nineteen months younger. The data was significant beyond one chance in a thousand by chance alone. Prof. John deCani, department chair of Statistics at Wharton, approved the research design and was very impressed with the data.

Then in the early 1990s, we tried the experiment another way; and again it was fortuitous that the group of patients we found to survey were older adults, thus continuing the factors that made the discovery easy to prove. We showed that the schizophrenics had the siblings less than two years younger, the psychotic depressed also had the siblings less than two years younger (mostly toward the end of that second year of life), and the nonpsychotic depressed had the sibling between two and three years younger. All studies reached beyond the .001 level of statistical significance.

Back to the Mechanisms

There are seven reasons why I believe the findings are correct.

1. It is a *loud noise* that precipitates the flashback to terrifying events associated with loud noises during war, and it is a *separation* from a most important person or group that precipitates the *initial* flashback to a separation trauma from infancy.
2. A person traumatized in combat returns to combat reality, experience and behavior, while the person traumatized during infancy returns to infant reality, experience and behavior.
3. When the person shifts to infant reality feelings and behavior, nearly everyone treats the patient as though he or she were an infant. In mental hospitals, art therapists bring crayons and coloring books for adult patients! Then they have movement therapy in which patients stand in a big circle and pass around a large yellow ball. Staff workers speak baby talk to the patients, often scolding them as if they were being naughty little children; but if the patients are good, they

are permitted to stay up an hour later at night. So this is really a preschool nursery environment. This way of relating to the patient confirms that at some level, *nearly everyone recognizes the patient has made a partial shift to infancy.* This treatment is counterproductive and keeps the patient locked into infant mind/brain/reality. It must not be permitted once the process is understood.

4. The fourth reason I believe the findings are correct is that after forty years of correlating reality and behavior with age at time of original trauma, I am able to determine clinically the age the original trauma occurred based on the behavior, reality, and feelings of the patient. This usually is confirmed if the history is known. When you can tell the patient the month of origin and then confirm the event that occurred at that time, it is convincing to the patient and helps the patient recognize and accept the origin and mechanism for the disorder. This is not difficult for a therapist to learn to do. Later, you will have an opportunity to test yourself on this ability.

5. Research surveys confirm the correlation between infant traumas in the first two years of life and the later development of schizophrenia and confirm a correlation between the same traumas in the next year of life and the later development of nonpsychotic depression. Every single study reached beyond the one chance in a thousand level of statistical significance.

6. The neurobiological changes we find in serious mental disorders, match very closely what we should *expect* to find with a shift in brain activity away from the later developmental brain structures to the earlier developmental structures that were active and developing at the time of the original trauma: We find hypertrophy of the structures that become more active (the brain stem increases in size, for example) and we find aberrant neuronal pathways developing *in between* structures that become more active (in the hippocampus, for example). Likewise, we find *disuse atrophy* in structures that become less active, and atrophy in their interconnecting pathways.

7. Not only is there a change in brain structure, chemistry and physiology reflecting the shift of activity to earlier developmental regions of the brain, but there also is a shift to a more immature level of function as measured on neuropsychological testing. And functions such as smooth eye pursuit return to what they were prior to their development.

Chapter 10

Other Searches for Cause

There have been numerous factors studied over the last century in hopes of finding the cause of schizophrenia, and we will mention some of these factors and consider their relative importance. Otherwise the reader might conclude we are unaware or simply missed some of the many other possible causes of schizophrenia.

The foregoing chapters are clear that it is highly unlikely for schizophrenia to occur without original trauma setting the stage for its later development, and without subsequent trauma sufficiently intense and similar to the first to activate the process later in life.

<u>Genetic Factors</u>

If the trauma-related findings are true—as I believe they are, to the best of my discernment—then any genetic weakness should be viewed as genetic predisposition. In other words, even if there is genetic predisposition, schizophrenia is highly unlikely to occur without original symptom-defining trauma and initial symptom-precipitating trauma.

I truly would like to know the extent of any genetic predisposition, but find it difficult in light of the methods of assessing genetic data. Some of the objections I have described in greater detail—*with references*—in the textbook *Delayed Posttraumatic Stress Disorders from Infancy: The Two Trauma Mechanism*.

I noted that genetic factors plus familial factors are combined and regarded as genetic. This leaves much room for distortion of findings. It is possible that most of what is called genetic might really be differences in child-rearing practices from one family tree to another. Or it might relate to hardships suffered by certain families. Even monkeys that suffer early separation are more prone to alcoholism, and that has nothing to do with genetics. Alcoholism might prevail in a family, and then the offspring will suffer numerous early separation traumas leading to more alcoholism and other serious disorders such as schizophrenia. Can we really call that genetic?

Because of the blending of genetic and familial factors, we really cannot tell what level of contribution is made by genetics alone; and regardless of whatever that contribution might be, the two traumas appear necessary in order to develop schizophrenia.

We must look further at the finding that siblings of a person with schizophrenia have an 8 percent chance of developing the disorder whereas nonidentical twins have a 12 percent chance of developing the disorder. This is strange because the genetic material of non-identical twins is no more alike than that of siblings who are not twins. This 50 percent increase therefore has *nothing* to do with genetics. But from the reporting of this data, we see there is another 50 percent inflation of data that is called genetic. That 50 percent probably relates to the fact that *some* of what happens to one twin is likely to happen to the other. If the mother is hospitalized for a month when one is fourteen months old, the other suffers the same separation at the same age. Yet this is mistakenly accepted as genetic.

Other studies report a 47 percent increase in schizophrenia among identical twins with schizophrenia as opposed to the 12 percent increase among nonidentical twins. This really sounds very impressive, but Dr. Robert Cancro, department chair of Psychiatry at the New York University Medical Center, noted that the concordance would be closer to 30 percent if one were to include the twins in whom both carry the gene but neither expresses it. That 30 percent gets reduced further because of the other reductions noted above.

Adding to those confounding factors are yet two more: identical twins are so much alike that they are more likely to be treated alike. Neither is fully unique. Also, each is attuned to the other's thoughts and feelings even at a distance. When one is upset, the other feels it. Why should these relationships not be factored in?

I am not attached to any particular result. I have always admired Albert Einstein's nonattachment to any particular finding or theory. Nonattachment is a true spiritual attribute. Einstein said that if everything he discovered was proven wrong, he would be happy to know it because he was searching only for truth. Though I may be dwarfed by the genius of Einstein, I have always felt compelled to emulate his devotion to science in a way that enables me to transcend my own opinions and beliefs in the search for truth. Mahatma Gandhi once said, "Truth, though spoken by one, is still truth"; and I am driven to know what it is!

The interpretation of genetic data so far does not make it possible for me to assess a genetic level of contribution to mental illness. At the present time, we have no way of knowing. My guess is that it represents a much smaller contribution than reports would lead us to believe. One thing is for sure, there is little that can be done about hereditary factors, other than decide not to have children or to take extra precautions to avoid infant trauma among those thought to be at genetic risk.

Contrast that with the finding that schizophrenia is a delayed posttraumatic stress disorder condition and therefore cannot occur without an original infant trauma. When the infant trauma of decades earlier no longer can be remembered or identified, we still have another clue as to origin, because the more recent event that precipitates the *initial* psychosis invariably is a separation trauma, not a loud noise—and the feelings, reality, and behavior, and even the neuroanatomic and neurobiological changes represent a partial return to the mind and brain of the infant.

I theorize that a genetic weakness might make it a little easier for the vulnerable person to develop a serious mental disorder. In some instances, it might even be a necessary factor in order for expression of the disorder. It still is not possible to have delayed PTSD without original trauma, but it certainly is possible to have delayed PTSD without genetic contribution. This will be whatever eventually is proven. I have no attachment to it being a large or a small contribution. This is for the geneticists to prove. Thus far, the percentage contribution has not been proven well enough to impress me one way or another; but truth ultimately rises to the surface, and eventually it will be established to everyone's satisfaction.

Second Trimester Factors

There have been extensive large-scale studies of these factors, but they account for only a very small contribution, and not a one-to-one ratio as with delayed PTSD. These factors include:

1. Starvation
2. Malnutrition
3. Paternal loss
4. Influenza virus

Starvation and malnutrition in the second trimester are factors that affect physical development of the fetus. They also affect the mother and her fears and worries and level of comfort. There is evidence that the fetus is very attuned to the mother—her thoughts, her feelings, and her fears. There even is evidence that it might be clairvoyant prior to birth, and this could be how the infant communicates and learns prior to spoken language development.

Here the confounding factors probably are more important: How secure is a mother with a small child after coming through the trauma of starvation? What happens in the next year or two of life? These are the kinds of questions that deserve closer scrutiny.

Loss of the Father

With paternal loss during the second trimester, the mother is upset during the pregnancy—which the fetus senses—but another confounding factor remains: How secure and happy is a mother with a new baby and no father to help provide for the family and rear the child? Is she still grieving? And is she now the breadwinner? These factors could result in infant separation trauma.

When large surveys are conducted, even a relatively minor contributing factor can be statistically significant. Then because it is a large-scale study, many equate the factor with being important, and it can gain wide recognition. This is misleading, because while it is significant as a result of the size of the survey, it can be relatively unimportant. We must not be fooled into equating large-scale, statistically significant data with being data of great importance. It still could be negligible.

Influenza Virus

Sarnoff Mednick of the University of Southern California surveyed huge populations of offspring of women who were in the second trimester of pregnancy during the 1957-1958 Asian flu epidemic to see if the flu virus correlated with the later development of schizophrenia. He found a positive correlation. But Timothy Crow of Oxford University then did a similar study and found no significance.

Many of the factors in the second trimester of pregnancy were searched with the thought that something happened to the development of the brain at that time based on postmortem studies of brains of persons with schizophrenia. This was studied without considering the possibility that brain changes could relate to shifting away from later developmental brain structures and reactivation of earlier developmental ones. It also was studied without the foreknowledge that stem cells do migrate and can regenerate damaged tissues in the brain.

Time of Year Born

Persons born late winter or early spring have an increased probability for developing schizophrenia. This is a consistent finding around the world that usually is attributed to viral infections, but represents a factor of only about 5 percent. In the late 1980s, when Dr. Wright and I surveyed a complete population of sixty people in two halfway houses and compared them to the first sixty "super normal" persons (who had full range of emotion; led active, productive lives; and had no history of mental illness), we found that five times as many in the disturbed group had a sibling born in the first eighteen months of life. The 5 percent related to time of year born pales by comparison to the *500 percent incidence* associated with the birth of a sibling within the first eighteen months of life that we found in our halfway house study—yet we hear only about the 5 percent change.

There are other explanations for the 5 percent: Holiday seasons cluster at certain times of the year, people get upset at holidays, and this can produce separation traumas depending on the age of the child at the holiday season when the mother becomes more upset. Thanksgiving, Christmas,

Hanukah, and New Years all cluster at the end of the year; and there are family gatherings at these times and people become upset, hospitals fill to capacity, and this produces more separation traumas in babies, especially if the mother is hospitalized. This data should be reviewed in light of the findings related to trauma. There might be more babies who are born in late winter/early spring who are at a peak age of origin for schizophrenia during that holiday season. Babies born in February and March would be nine to eleven months old during the first holiday season, and twenty-one to twenty-three months old during their next holiday season.

The data south of the equator is supposed to be the same however, and their seasons are just the opposite months of the year. This requires further review. Only 10 percent of the world's population lives south of the equator, and I have not reviewed the data south of the equator.

Nonetheless, even if it represents a 5 percent increase, this pales by comparison to the *five-fold* incidence of schizophrenia among those with a sibling less than nineteen months younger. The change in incidence related to a more severe trauma, such as the death of the mother during the same age interval, should be far greater still.

Other Siblings

There also is an increase in schizophrenia among those who have a sibling less than two years older (Westergaard and Mortensen, Archives of General Psychiatry, 1999;56:993-998). This is understandable because an older sibling would still be more demanding of its mother's attention because of its threat of separation, but this data is not as useful as birth of a younger sibling because it does not pinpoint a specific age of origin.

The greatest increase in schizophrenia was found in a positive correlation between the number of older siblings and the incidence of schizophrenia. Westergaard and Mortensen pinned their hopes on this proving a viral etiology. When I questioned Westergaard, she wrote that they only were searching for viral etiology even though the study mathematically was supposed to be able to identify all possible causes.

Years earlier, I had written about the older sibling in the textbook and noted that if an older sibling were seriously injured or dying, it might require all the mother's attention, *and if there are five older siblings, there is five times the chance of this occurring.* This certainly would account for the positive correlation with the *number* of older siblings. Westergaard and Mortensen concluded that the cause was viral because with a larger number of older siblings, there was a greater chance of one bringing home a virus. This does not explain why the birth of a *younger* sibling in the first two years of life leads to an increase in schizophrenia; it does not explain the age-of-origin symptom specificity, which correlates with an age-specific separation trauma, and it does not explain the subsequent initial symptom-*precipitating* trauma being a separation. Their study lacks in-depth understanding necessary to decipher the data. This is not meant as a criticism of them. No one else at the time knew of the separation trauma findings either. Westergaard and Mortensen are honest, sincere, and energetic in their research. I appreciated their supplying me with data that I could not have gathered otherwise. The data has been very helpful.

If the study did not include all kinds of separation traumas at specific ages, how would it ever identify such rare separation traumas as the barn burning down and killing all the cows? These rare separation traumas were identified by *first identifying clinically the age of origin* of the disorder and then searching for what trauma occurred at that particular month. Such understanding could be helpful for conducting large studies in the future.

Obstetric and Birth Traumas

These and other traumas—which occur prior to the separation trauma that sets the stage for the later development of schizophrenia—serve as *antecedent* traumas, which intensify the separation traumas that follow. Throughout the posttraumatic stress disorder literature, it is reported that posttraumatic stress disorder is cumulative. Each successive trauma adds to previous ones. Freud even reported this about war neuroses in 1926, stating that it was more pronounced among those who previously had more anxiety.

In catatonic schizophrenia, a near-death struggle at birth might serve as the original symptom-defining trauma; but in other categories of schizophrenia, birth trauma is only an antecedent trauma.

Stress Factors

If there is increased stress at the time of the initial trauma, that trauma is experienced as more severe. The stress can be physical, chemical, or any kind of environmental stress. Likewise, excessive stress later in life can contribute to the intensity of the subsequent trauma that precipitates the return to the earlier gestalt. This too can be physical, chemical, environmental, situational, financial, metabolic, nutritional, viral, or anything else that produces too much stress.

Migration

A number of studies report higher incidence of schizophrenia among groups of people who migrate from one location to another. These studies do not explore the separation traumas that the infant experiences in the first two years of life. Such traumas might include physical separation from familiar surroundings, emotional separation from mother when she is preoccupied with finding a home or food for the family or when she senses a feeling of alienation and nonacceptance in the new community to which she has moved.

Without understanding the original symptom-defining trauma and initial symptom-precipitating trauma in delayed posttraumatic stress disorder and the two-trauma mechanism, these studies are destined to fall short of the mark because the researchers do not know where to search for cause.

Elusiveness of Separation Traumas

Furthermore, separation trauma eludes researchers because it is not one event or one particular trauma that sets the stage for the later development of the disorder: the traumas include anything that can cause the infant to experience a threat of separation. Researchers also dilute their findings many fold by not being aware of an age-of-origin specificity for symptoms and diagnostic categories. Thus they might try to correlate the incidence of schizophrenia or depression with a specific trauma over the first twenty years of life instead of the more narrow age range-of-origin of specific symptoms.

There is variability caused by a myriad of circumstances and differences in child-rearing practices. This can be confusing and cloud the picture, but among all these variables, there are common denominators related to the age-of-origin specificities.

The Original Symptom-defining Trauma

The original infant separation traumas that set the stage for delayed posttraumatic stress disorder include, but are not limited to, the following:

1. Moving to new house—mother busies herself making it look like home
2. Birth of a sibling—mother is away for five days prior to returning with new baby (especially traumatic in previous generations because of better bonding followed by longer separation)
3. Older sibling becomes very sick and might have a terminal illness that requires all of mother's attention (the more older siblings there are, the more likely this is to occur)
4. Death of parent—mother is grieving and emotionally unavailable if father dies
5. Father causes mother to be upset (is alcoholic, has an affair, quits his job)
6. Mother is alcoholic, depressed, or upset—causing emotional separation
7. *Thousands* of other events, conditions, or circumstances, which upset the mother and cause the infant to experience a threat of separation

Note: *Mothers are most important to the baby in the first three years of life.* With all, or nearly all mammalian infants, it is the mother that rears the baby. Women are more right brain oriented and men more left brain oriented. This right brain function is more intuitive and is required for knowing what the baby wants and needs. Brain imaging studies reveal that the right orbital and right prefrontal cortex of the mother interacts with the right orbital and right prefrontal cortex of the infant in rhythmical fashion, and this is how the limbic system develops. Just observe any woman picking up a baby in a social setting and making all kinds of sounds and gestures that men would have great difficulty duplicating. Very few men could do this. Their role in early infant trauma is when they cause the mother to be upset and do not provide for her a safe, comfortable, and secure environment with lots of emotional support.

The Initial Symptom-precipitating Trauma

In serious mental and emotional disorders, the second trauma in the two-trauma mechanism is a separation from a "most important person" in the present (husband, wife, girlfriend, boyfriend, or group) whether real, imagined, anticipated, or implied. Even a terrible failure in one's life can cause a person to *anticipate* rejection by loved ones.

Stress Factors

These cause the second trauma to be more severe, and can include financial, nutritional, environmental, metabolic, viral, and anything else that produces stress. Many of the same stress factors can also intensify the original symptom-defining trauma.

Facilitating Factors

Drugs and alcohol can serve as grease in the mechanism and thereby facilitate the initial onset of schizophrenia or other serious disorders. Without the abusive substance, the disorder might never occur.

Perpetuating Factors

These are factors that cause the original infant trauma to remain activated after initial onset of illness. They include continued rejection, failure, toxic relationships, and even interaction with family. These will be discussed in later chapters, which describe treatment and elimination of the perpetuating factors.

Biological Change

Biological change is viewed largely as the result of the disease process and not the cause. Nearly every biological change is precisely what one should expect to find with a sudden shift of brain activity away from the adult brain structures and into the areas of brain that were active and developing at the precise time of the original trauma during infancy. Some change might be set in motion by the original trauma, but most occurs later as a result of this shift in areas of brain activity and the return of the overwhelming fears from the earlier time. These changes are described in greater detail in the paper *The Unification Model for Mental Illness* (See Appendix).

Chapter 11

Age of Origin of Other Symptoms and Diagnostic Categories

Since posttraumatic stress disorder is fueled by a primal instinct for survival, which applies to all species all the time, and since this instinct protects us not only from death, but protects us from unpleasant thoughts and feelings, it is likely that the delayed posttraumatic stress disorder mechanism applies to all or nearly all mental and emotional disorders and is the major mechanism for illness in many of them.

We will examine a few in this chapter, including schizophrenia, depression, ADHD, school violence, autism, symbiosis, drug and alcohol dependence, bipolar disorders, borderline personality disorder, eating disorders, and more.

These are shown to follow a delayed posttraumatic stress disorder pattern, with the exception of autism and symbiosis, which—to the extent they relate to infant separation trauma—represent acute instead of delayed type posttraumatic stress disorder.

Autism

Autism spectrum disorders can occur with acute trauma. This is not a large part of my practice; but I have seen at least six infants who, at about fifteen months of age, suddenly stopped talking immediately following a terrible traumatic experience, such as a car accident in which the mother is screaming and bleeding. Many others with autism spectrum disorder had mothers who were mentally or emotionally disturbed, traumatized by divorce, or were drug addicted when their affected children were infants. I also saw two who had early separation traumas but also had very high levels of heavy metal toxicity as determined by hair analysis. These were the only two I tested for heavy metals.

Forty years ago, the ratio of autistic boys to autistic girls was ten to one. I attributed this ratio to one trauma boys had that girls did not, namely, circumcision without anesthesia and without the mother present. This points to a very early age of origin. The ten to one ratio shifted in recent years to only three or four autistic boys to one autistic girl, and no one noticed. Thus the recent many fold increase in autism, mathematically, represents an increase primarily in non gender-specific autism. This increase must be something that affects infant boys and girls alike, such as mercury and other toxins in our environment or the advent of the working mother.

With careful examination of data, we should find a shift in the kinds of autism found, because the increase likely includes a shift to a later average age-of-origin instead of mostly at circumcision.

Mercury is a powerful neurotoxin and can have a profound affect on the brain. We have seen that stress factors can increase the intensity of any trauma and mercury produces stress. A physician friend reported three young children in one family developing autism within the same two weeks of receiving their vaccinations. Even if autism were as common as one chance in one hundred, for three out of three to develop autism would mean a very high level of statistical significance.

The advent of the working mother also affects boys and girls alike, and we know the impact of separation trauma on the infant and the toddler. It is the advent of the working mother that might be the leading cause for—what some believe to be—a twenty-fold increase in autism.

This concept is unpopular because it is taken as an indictment of modern-day mothers. Thus, as with schizophrenia, depression, ADHD, and other serious disorders, no one has conducted the obvious study to check the incidence among offspring of working versus nonworking mothers.

This broad range for autism, from the age of circumcision to eighteen months of life, eventually should reveal age-of-origin specificities for the various symptoms and types of autism that might relate to trauma. Perhaps all that will be required for this purpose is simple survey data. Few, if any, suspect this possible origin however; and many would not participate in this area of study because it would be unpopular and might draw criticism.

In June 2007, I attended an autism lecture given by a professor from the Yale Child Study Center who had conducted extensive autism research. I was hopeful of valuable new information. Some of the data was informative, but I was disappointed to find the same level of understanding that existed decades earlier for schizophrenia. He was convinced the cause was neurobiological because of the many brain changes—even though there is not one shred of evidence that shows the changes are the cause instead of the result of a psychological process—and he was convinced that it is hereditary because some families have several autistic children. Again, he failed to differentiate between familial and hereditary.

The professor was highly credentialed and very much esteemed by the psychoanalytic group that invited him to speak. While I found it incredible that he did not consider the possibility that biological change might be the result and not the cause of the disorder and that he automatically decided the disorder must be genetic because he found some families with a number of autistic children, *the real shock came when he asserted that we must not consider early trauma because this might be viewed as blaming the parent*—which, when understood, it does not.

Science is open exploration, without preconceived notions and without excluding areas of investigation. I take time to review the work of this current leader in the field, just to illustrate that what is politically correct or most popular might have little to do with science or with truth. Years earlier, I was stunned to hear a well-known schizophrenia researcher also say publicly that he would *not dare* do a survey that might correlate schizophrenia with infant separation trauma.

The unspoken remainder of that statement, of course, is "even if doing so might lead to prevention and treatment of mental illness."

It is essential that we not just remain vigilant and examine carefully the credentials determined by man but we also must search deeply for truth. It is easy to win quick recognition in the mental health field through finding answers that people want to hear. Perhaps this is why many researchers in the field have been led so far astray. Another factor is the art of influencing outcome studies—which has been mastered by industry and special interests for commercial gain.

This same phenomenon was described thousands of years ago in Scriptures, where it tells how we are led astray from truth by needs or desires for worldly things or pleasures. In the same text we are given safeguards for preventing such pitfalls.

How simple it would be to compare the incidence of autism among offspring of working versus nonworking mothers! When adjusted for the incidence of other traumas—i.e., by eliminating those with other known traumas during the first eighteen months of life—we could isolate further the impact caused by the working mother.

Symbiosis

In my practice, I only had one case of symbiosis, but had seen dozens of cases of symbiosis in my training at the Eastern Pennsylvania Psychiatric Institute prior to uncovering the delayed posttraumatic stress disorder mechanism. These children are most unusual in their clinging to mother, and if mother is not present, they will cling to their chair, and if they move to another chair, they will dart to the other chair and immediately cling to it.

The one case—which Bruno Bettelheim and I both evaluated—had a specific age of origin of twenty-one months when the mother was raped in front of the family at gunpoint and immediately became acutely psychotic. I never knew if it were that trauma that caused the child's symbiosis or whether it was compounded afterward by the mother clinging to the child like a frightened child clinging to a doll.

Bruno Bettelheim and I corresponded for a while after we did the evaluation. It is interesting that he thought the age of origin of autism was the first eighteen months of life and that Margaret Mahler said the age of origin of childhood schizophrenia was in the first eighteen months of life. Both are right; but what neither realized is that autism might represent acute posttraumatic stress disorder, which later becomes chronic, and schizophrenia represents the delayed type with multiple recurrent psychotic episodes.

Symptom Expression

There are countless possible factors involved in symptom formation, *but it is the age of origin that provides the common denominator.* This determines the region of brain that is reactivated and also provides the basis for age-of-origin specificities related to feelings, behavior, reality, body movements, and level of affective expression.

Psychosomatic medicine recognizes a similar phenomenon: the same stress can cause a great variety of disorders. In one person it might cause ulcers, in another it can produce a skin reaction, and in still another the same stress might result in tension headaches or high blood pressure. Likewise, early trauma can set the stage for a variety of symptom expression, but the symptoms still will have an underlying common denominator based on age-of-origin specificity.

Not all symptoms have to be present at the same time. Regression is not even across the board, and only a narrow band of the earlier mind/brain/reality might be present. A patient might exhibit a single symptom from an earlier time. For example, a man might fly a jet airplane, be a world-class chess champion, have a socially acceptable demeanor, and yet experience that he is being controlled by radio waves. This particular reality has its origin between thirteen and fifteen months when the infant experiences most acutely that everything it does is monitored and controlled.

For some psychological problems, we have data that identifies a precise peak age-of-origin and age range-of-origin; and for other disorders, we can only estimate based on the five recognized parameters we use (feelings, behavior, reality, body movements, and level of affective expression). Some parameters are well established, but others need more data for confirmation. Birth-of-a-sibling trauma provides easy access to age-of-origin specificity from age one to three, but data is not as readily available for the first year of life.

Differences in Symptoms Related to Child-rearing Practices

It is easy to search birth-of-a-sibling trauma and find that different symptoms and diagnostic categories correspond with different ages at time of birth of a sibling. This requires correlating symptoms with one trauma at a precise, known age during infancy. It is more difficult to determine symptom variation that corresponds with different child-rearing practices because there are as many differences in child rearing as there are families.

These differences produce symptom variation nonetheless, but not the same clear common denominators. The data is researchable, but will require much larger studies.

In some families, a child who is traumatized during the age range-of-origin for paranoid schizophrenia might have been reared in a crib, so the mother did not have to watch him and follow him everywhere he went. Only detailed histories on larger numbers of persons with schizophrenia will tell us whether that person would have a greater propensity to develop undifferentiated instead of paranoid schizophrenia. Undifferentiated schizophrenia probably has an origin within the age rage-of-origin of paranoid schizophrenia, but we do not have enough data on that category to make an accurate age range-of-origin determination.

There can be differences based on quality of mothering and quality of bonding. This actually can have an inverse effect in relation to some serious mental disorders because separation following good bonding is more traumatic. Nonetheless, it is better to have good bonding and then avoid early separation trauma.

Some of the differences in symptom expression relate to the impact on a baby of a mother being away from eight to five every day and then coming home to another full-time job versus a mother suddenly being away completely for five days, or leaving for a month; and these differ still when the baby is in pain and extremely distressed during the time she is away.

What is the impact on the baby if it is left in the care of a grandmother in the same house or in a different house; or left with a stranger in the same house or with a stranger in a different house; or in a daycare center, especially during the age of stranger anxiety; or with a series of babysitters in a series of different houses? These questions must be researched and answered for each particular age of infant and with considerations of prior bonding and prior traumas.

One young lady asked me to endorse the cover of her book on how to select the very best babysitter. She really loved her children and wanted the very best for them, which is why the outcome was so tragic. She thought she was doing the best for them by carefully screening the babysitters. She was an expert because she hired a series of more than two dozen babysitters and really knew how to choose one. I told her the best babysitter is the one she sees when she looks in the mirror. Unfortunately, my comments came too late for her and her children and for the talk shows where she soared to popularity because she said what people wanted to hear. Three years later, she called. Her younger child was hospitalized with manic psychosis and her older one was caught making bombs.

Infant traumas will have variation in results. This is no different than with PTSD from adult life. For example, in an airplane crash in Managua, Nicaragua, a Boeing 737 struck the runway at a sharp angle, tore off a wing, spun down the runway at 161 mph, and crashed into trees. The smell of jet fuel was everywhere, and all the lights were out. The escape chutes did not function, people had difficulty exiting, and they were terrified of being engulfed in flames.

Months later, some had flashbacks at the smell of gasoline, others at the sound of a loud noise, some at riding in a fast-moving vehicle, others were frightened of the dark, still others had a fear of being in an enclosed space, and one was afraid to jump into a swimming pool because he was terrified when he had to jump off the wing of the airplane, not knowing how far it was to the ground because it was too dark to see.

From the PTSD literature, we know that the reactions of the victims also varied according to their previous traumas and the age and gender of each individual. There are millions of possible variables that cause each person to re-experience the trauma differently, but all individuals do return precisely to that moment of trauma.

When the trauma occurs during infancy and early childhood, there are specific age-of-origin markers along with the variations caused by differences in child-rearing practices.

<u>Test Yourself on Age-of-origin Specificities</u>

Sometimes pondering a simple question will lead to a revelation of an age-old mystery. Consider the mystery of schizophrenia.

With all the billions of dollars spent on the search for cause—including chemical imbalances and differences in neuroanatomy, neurotransmission, time of year born, viral infections, migration, starvation, and events occurring during the second trimester of pregnancy—with all this and with the mountains of peer-reviewed literature reference the search for cause, no one had identified a cause that applies to all schizophrenia; and without which, schizophrenia is unlikely to occur. There are amazing findings *about* schizophrenia; yet nothing that identifies cause, and without identifying the cause, how is it possible to prevent? Further, without understanding the cause, on what can we base our approach to treatment?

Let us step aside from the vast number of studies and findings and ask a few simple questions that you yourself will be able to determine, even without extensive training or experience. Test yourself and see if you can determine the age-of-origin of the following symptoms:

1. In catatonic schizophrenia, a person often holds one posture for days at a time without moving, and then suddenly erupts in a violent thrusting motion of the body as if in a life-and-death struggle.

When is the only time in one's life cycle that this can occur? This one is easy. Think about it for a minute. When does a person hold one body posture for days at a time?

When phrased this way, the answer is all but obvious even though no one in the field has identified it yet. This occurs only once in our life cycle. It is prior to birth, coupled with a near-death struggle to exit the birth canal. We don't have data on this, just observations, but it seems to be what the body movements are depicting in catatonic schizophrenia. Furthermore, this used to be one of the most common forms of schizophrenia one hundred years ago, and now it is relatively uncommon. It makes sense that modern obstetrics has eliminated most of the near-death experience at birth, and thereby all but eliminated catatonic schizophrenia.

Note: No amount of money studying brain, genetics, and chemistry would arrive at this simple answer. Let's test ourselves with a couple more examples.

2. A family brought in a twenty-year-old man who was convinced he never would be able to walk again because his feet hurt. The reality that he never would be able to walk was more real to him than the reality that he had just walked into my office. He literally was locked in an earlier part of the mind and brain that was experiencing everyone else could walk but he could not, and he was experiencing pain when he placed his feet on the ground.

I pondered, what age would a healthy young person experience most intensely the reality that everyone else can walk but he cannot? By asking this simple question, the answer again becomes obvious. Before the baby takes its first steps, it looks around and notices that everyone else can walk but it cannot. And the symptom of feet hurting takes us to the same age because it corresponds with a baby placing all its weight on one foot for the first time.

So I said to this family, "Something happened when he was just twelve months old." They said nothing happened. I insisted it did, they insisted it didn't. Finally, I said, "Something happened to cause *his mother* to be *extremely upset* when he was just twelve months old!" This jostled memories, and one recalled the patient had a brother who died when the patient was just twelve months old! Can you imagine the grief reaction in the mother? Emotionally, her mind no longer was on her twelve-month-old baby.

I further told them that in order to have the breakdown now, there also had to be a separation from some other most important person in the present. They revealed that his girlfriend left him one month before the bizarre symptoms appeared.

Test yourself on a third patient:

3. Another family brought in a young man who hung his mother's cat because it was answering the telephone. At what age would a man experience most intensely the reality that cats and dogs can talk? Think for a minute. This is not difficult.

Obviously, this occurs after he learns to say a few words, but before he realizes that meowing or barking are not part of our language. So I told the family that something happened when he was fourteen months old. I then learned that he had a sister born when he was just fourteen months old.

See how easy this is? Why wouldn't a therapist's first question be "Where did that reality come from? or "When during infancy is that real to a person?"

Many in the profession are so influenced by the glitz of fancy research equipment, the influence of volumes of peer-reviewed journal articles, and the marketing of the new drugs that their only questions might be "What is the diagnosis?" and "What medications do we have to treat this diagnosis?"

Regardless of one's belief system, there are profound truths, written thousands of years ago, which seem to apply today:

Isaiah wrote: "Therefore, behold, I will proceed to do a marvelous work among this people, even a marvelous work and a wonder: for the wisdom of their wise men shall perish, and the understanding of the intelligent shall be hid." Paul wrote: "God chose the ignorant of the world so that He would put the wise to shame, and God chose the weak ones of the world so that He would shame the strong, and God chose the lowly of the world, even those who were despised, even the things that were nothing, so that He would make ineffective the things that were."

I haven't figured if I am weak, ignorant, lowly, or despised; but I see truth in what was revealed to me. I take credit only for the errors in this book, and I am humbled when I look back over the last several decades and realize how long it took me to recognize the validity of what has been there all the time, just waiting for someone to grasp.

Chapter 12

Age of Origin of Other Delayed Posttraumatic Stress Disorders

<u>Borderline personality disorder</u> could have its origin as early as the first two weeks of life. Dr. Gerald E. Davidson, psychiatrist at Élan One in Maine, reported in 1985 that out of 160 mostly borderline adolescents, 35% were adopted. In a personal interview, he said most of these were adopted in the first two weeks of life. When compared to the 2% adopted in the overall population, that is hugely significant.

Students at the Élan One boarding school/treatment center were from wealthy families, which perhaps allowed for the earlier age at time of adoption. In the same year, 25% of the borderline patients at the Institute for Living in Hartford were adopted, and the Institute's survey of other area hospitals including West Chester, and also adolescents at Chestnut Lodge, revealed 25% of their borderline patients also were adopted. The age of adoption was not reported for these, but most would have had very early separation traumas, with foster care and then later adoptions. The statistical significance warrants close and careful scrutiny.

In Child Trend's 1985 survey of 15,416 adopted children, 42% of the twelve- to seventeen-year-olds who were adopted after twelve months (forty-seven children) had seen a psychotherapist as opposed to 5.1% of those reared by both biological parents. The significance of this emphasizes the critical importance of avoiding early separation traumas.

Sadly, the very ones in charge of adoption seem to be unaware of the magnitude of the above findings. Nine months should be adequate time to find an appropriate adoptive family. Finding just the right family, who meets all the demographics, serves little purpose after a child has been severely and permanently damaged by one or more untimely separations. The baby needs a mother, one mother, who will love and care for it from birth.

<u>Unintentional Abuse at the Hands of Adoption and Child Protection Agencies</u>

Adoption agencies, acting in accordance with federally mandated guidelines, often delay adoptions for lengthy periods of time while they continue to do their job. A national survey shows that only two percent of babies are adopted in the first year of life, and another 44 percent between ages one through five. If the harmful and enduring effects of early separation traumas were recognized, this would not be tolerated for any reason.

If federal regulating agencies were aware of the high incidence of specific damage caused by separation trauma at each particular month, they would realize that the nine months of pregnancy must suffice as adequate time to find adoptive parents. Adoption at birth, however, could cause adoption agencies to have a conflict of interest, because much of their work might be eliminated.

Child protection agencies, in particular, need education and training that is not available to them. The bureaucratic and judicial systems are so entrenched that no one is able to hear anything outside the system's status quo. Therefore training in this area is hardly ever a consideration among the bureaucratic hierarchy, and the children they are supposed to protect are being exposed to potential harm.

Early separations can lead to borderline personality disorder, and conduct, identity, impulse and substance abuse disorders. Just a five-day separation in the first 18 months of life resulted in a five-fold incidence of schizophrenia in our studies on schizophrenia. This was studying just one of the many infant separation traumas. There is a similar increase in schizoaffective disorder, bipolar disorder and psychotic depression over the next six months, and a similar increase in nonpsychotic depression over the following ten months. The Child Trend data (Zill, 1985) revealed an eight-fold incidence of need for psychotherapy in the first 17 years of life among adopted children. Quite possibly there would be no increase in need for psychotherapy if the babies were adopted at birth.

During the past 20 years, I have seen numerous examples of babies taken from mothers for reasons that appear only to serve the needs of the agencies. Some mothers were in treatment with me, and I knew them to be fully capable of caring for their children. The most likely purpose I could imagine for snatching the baby from the mother was to gain control over the mother and compel her to attend their prescribed classes, while keeping the babies for months and even for years at a time. Such procedures, of course, nurture the enrollment goals of the agencies that provide the training, but often at a high and irreversible cost of psychological damage to the children involved.

Nonetheless, the courts are prone to endorse the recommendations of these organizations, often ignoring the recommendations of true experts in the field.

Perhaps calling attention to this will cause the agencies to scrutinize their practices more carefully, and alert others to be aware of them too. What a merciful gift this would be to the untold numbers of children waiting to be helped!

<u>Disorganized Schizophrenia</u>

For many years, I suspected that the age of origin of disorganized schizophrenia—formerly known as hebephrenic schizophrenia—would peak at about eight to nine months, the age of stranger anxiety. This is prior to the birth of a sibling, and therefore data is not as readily available. Finally I encountered a recovered person with classical disorganized type schizophrenia. He had extremely bizarre delusions and hallucinations. History revealed that his mother was hospitalized for a month when he was *eight months old*.

<u>Rage</u>

To illustrate a difference in symptom expression, let us compare the above eight-to-nine-month separation case to the Unabomber who sent letter bombs to persons across the country. He was hospitalized when he was nine months old, and his mother was allowed to see him, but only through a glass partition.

Rage is proportionate to helplessness, and no one is as helpless as a baby when the mother is not there. The Unabomber was physically very ill, could see his mother, but could not be comforted by her. Even she attributes his later violence to that separation. Since the mother is the whole world to the infant, the rage is directed outward to the whole world. Forty years later, when a lady friend left him, he returned to the earlier separation and no longer could function well enough to teach math at Harvard. Instead, he holed up in the woods and sent bombs indiscriminately to others. While the infant mind directed rage outward to the whole world, the adult mind attempted to justify the murderous actions by finding specific reasons to kill certain individuals he did not know.

The research, once more, is very simple. Can you imagine the billions it would cost to check brain chemistries, microscopic details of brains of deceased violent versus peaceable individuals, and PET scans comparing differences, and then the genetic research studies?

By contrast, a study to identify the origin of such murderous rage, indiscriminately directed outward toward all people, would not be difficult *because we know where to look*. Check the early histories of one hundred of the most violent criminals for incidence of infant separation traumas in the first two years of life and compare that to early histories of one hundred of the most peaceable individuals. With more cumulative data, a peak age-of-origin and age range-of-origin also will emerge and eventually the severity of each type of separation trauma.

Data is available for any of these studies as soon as there are funds for this work because many women have served in the military, and the precise date when they spent two weeks in basic training is known and recorded. We should find a continuum of mental and emotional disorders dependent strictly on the age in months of the infant when the mother was sent away.

School Violence

This operates according to the same mechanism. When the mother is sick or incapacitated, all the baby can do is scream to vent its rage. Place that rage in an adult body with a brilliant mind and access to automatic weapons, teach it to use those weapons—through daily TV violence—and the unthinkable can occur.

There has been a marked increase in school violence in recent decades. The shootings at Littleton High School shocked the world. When rejected by classmates, the two children returned to early rage and fired automatic weapons, spraying bullets indiscriminately at everyone and ultimately killing themselves.

Emotions are more intense than thoughts, and while the assailants would not remember the earlier trauma, murderous rage from infancy resurfaced and sixteen died, with twenty-three more injured. Shortly thereafter, another child in Atlanta—who had just been jilted by his girlfriend—took the step back in time and shot seven more children in his classroom. Both cases followed the pattern of separation or rejection precipitating the return to an earlier time.

Many point to the increase in television violence as being responsible for the increase in school violence, but this is not the cause. Both the school violence *and* the increased interest in violence displayed on TV more likely relate to the advent of the working mother in America. They also relate to the increase in divorce, the changing of values in our society and the falling away from the teaching of sound, moral and spiritual principles in the home and in school.

Help is available. The fact that you worked when your children were infants does not mean that they are going to take guns to school and shoot people; but depending on the amount of frustration and rage they experienced during early infancy, there is an increased potential for violent behavior, especially when rejected by teachers or other children.

Adolf Hitler and Saddam Hussein

Adolf Hitler had a horrible infancy. His mother had lost her first three children to diphtheria, all within a two-month period just prior to becoming pregnant with Adolf, and she was in a terrible abusive relationship. Saddam Hussein also experienced early separation traumas. His father left his mother six months prior to Saddam's birth, and then shortly thereafter, his thirteen-year-old brother died of cancer. This left his mother severely depressed; and Saddam, as an infant, was sent to the family of his maternal uncle until he was three.

The Washington DC Sniper

When the DC snipers were on the loose, I profiled one on Fox national TV and said we would find an early separation trauma followed by a more recent separation from some other most important person. Later we learned that the elder shooter's mother had died of cancer when he was three. His rage was of an age prior to three, but his mother probably learned of the cancer long before she died, which would have produced an earlier emotional separation. His trauma had to be very early because the rage was directed out to the whole world. The victims included men, women, children, and people of all races. After he was caught, we also learned that, indeed, he did have a subsequent separation from his wife and children.

Such violence and murderous rage can be prevented by minimizing early separation traumas and not frustrating the baby's early needs. The most important thing a mother can teach a child is how to love, because the byproduct of love is happiness. This helps the child to have a happy life and be a blessing to society.

Social Factors Leading to Infant Separation

There is another reason why infants have been traumatized in recent decades. This is one of the most unfortunate mistakes of the last century, and it was an innocent mistake, not intended to harm. One of the most noted and respected child development experts in the country—who was a *pediatrician* and not a child psychoanalyst—recommended that mothers stay home with their babies for the first four months because it is hard for the *mother* to give up the baby any sooner!

This is the message the public wanted to hear. It meant more money for the family, more luxuries, more tax dollars for the politicians, and fewer smelly diapers to change. Anyone who advocates for working mothers wins favor in the news.

Contrary to what the noted pediatrician recommended, Rene Spitz reported in the *Psychoanalytic Study of the Child*, volume 1, 1945 that after good bonding in the first four to six months of life, separation from mother is far more traumatic.

While the working mother has been viewed as a financial necessity, this concept undoubtedly has caused instead an economic drain on family and nation because of cost of treatment, loss of productivity, human suffering, and even loss of lives.

Prospective studies will do little to identify the cause of violence. To gather data on one hundred children, from birth through adolescence, who would take a gun to school and shoot other children, might require gathering data on a million children to find the one hundred. That would be unwieldy and cost-prohibitive. This is why I would choose a retrospective study of one hundred of the most violent children in America and review their early backgrounds (first two years of life) for infant separation trauma, and then compare that to the early backgrounds of one hundred of the most peaceable children in America. This way we can study fewer and yet have conclusive results, *within months*, because we know where to look.

Paranoid Schizophrenia

The age range-of-origin of paranoid delutions is mostly between twelve and twenty-one months. When the infant begins to walk, the whole world—which to the infant is the mother—watches and follows it everywhere it goes. With trauma after first learning to walk followed by separation trauma later in life, persons can re-experience the early reality that everyone is watching and following them everywhere they go.

In general, the earlier the age of origin, the more bizarre the symptoms. Paranoia from age twenty-one months might be "Those people over there are talking about me." At age seventeen months, it more likely is "They are talking about me on television;" and at thirteen to fifteen months, it might be "Aliens have implanted something in my brain and are monitoring and controlling everything I do." In previous generations, this was radio waves or a criminal gang or a machine controlling them—depending on the theme of the day. At thirteen to fifteen months, the infant experiences most intensely the reality that everything is monitored and controlled. As soon as it is wet, the diaper is changed; when it is hungry, it is fed; when teething, it is given a pacifier. It is picked up and put in a high chair, picked up and put in a car seat, picked up and put in a crib, etc. Everything is monitored and controlled.

Let's move up to the age-of-origin of the former diagnosis of simple schizophrenia. These people are unique in that they become world travelers and keep returning to the *mother*land. I only evaluated three where I could determine the age of origin, and these were three who had a sibling born at seventeen months. That's the age when the toddler is wandering into the next room and peeking back around the corner to see if the mother is still there.

More affect begins to creep in with trauma subsequent to that time. Perhaps prior to eighteen months, more of the infants are so traumatized that they simply become numb. In daycare centers, this might be considered good adjustment because the baby no longer cries.

Schizoaffective disorder, bipolar hypomanic disorder, and psychotic depression have an age range-of-origin mostly between twenty and twenty-four months—with overlap, but in that order. Bipolar hypomania peaks at twenty-two months. If you have someone with this disorder and there is another child less than three years younger, check the birth dates—it nearly always will be twenty-two months younger.

I do not have sufficient data on patients with manic-type bipolar disorder. This work has never enjoyed the charitable donation of a single penny; it has relied upon observations, national databases, mathematical calculations, the help of friends who gathered additional data, and data gathered on a few large-scale studies that others were kind enough to provide.

In terms of the psychoses, I have not yet encountered one with a known age-of-origin subsequent to twenty-four months. Asthma peaks at twenty-four months, nonpsychotic depression is between twenty-four and thirty-four months, and twenty-six to twenty-seven months correlates with the most intense self-condemnation and suicidal depression. I recognized this for twenty-five years before I understood why. Toilet training on average is accomplished by two years and three months. Few appreciate how terrible the toddler can feel when everyone else can poop in the potty and it cannot. When traumatized at this age, and later traumatized by another separation that is sufficiently intense and similar to the first, the symptoms of extreme self-condemnation and suicidal depression are difficult to miss.

Any student of mental illness knows that suicide among persons with schizophrenia is impulsive, whereas suicide with the nonpsychotic depressed is planned. Why should this be so? The answer is simple once we realize the age of origin of each. Schizophrenia has its origin in the first two years of life—which is prior to toilet training. Impulse control begins with toilet training. This is the first time a baby struggles to control a bodily impulse. Most <u>nonpsychotic depression</u> has its origin after the baby has gained some bodily control.

Thus, with schizophrenia, suicide is, "Have the thought, cut the wrist;" "Have the thought, pull the trigger;" "Have the thought, swallow the pills." This is because toilet training and impulse control are learned after the age of origin of schizophrenia. With nonpsychotic depression, it's "Have the thought, think about it, plan it, and do it."

<u>Attention deficit hyperactivity disorder (ADHD)</u> has its origin in the first two years of life. The massive increase most likely correlates with the advent of the working mother in America. The disorder can be acute or delayed type. The toddler is in constant motion and is traumatized when the mother starts to work. In the delayed type PTSD, the child can return to the earlier hyperactivity when it separates from home to start school. This causes a partial return to being in constant motion. There also is very little impulse control—which further identifies the age-of-origin as being prior to twenty-four months—and the brain weight is less, which is consistent with other disorders of early origin such as schizophrenia.

Here again we could study genetics, biochemistry, anatomical changes in brain structure, and areas of increased or diminished brain activity, spending billions of dollars and discovering many new things. While this would provide new information, it would not bring us closer to cause and therefore could not lead to primary prevention.

Physical factors also can play a role in this disorder and should be studied. These include diet, mineral depletion, and chemical sensitivities to airborne toxins. Many children who are given this diagnosis have hypoglycemia instead. The average child now consumes up to forty-eight teaspoons of sugar each day. A Coke and a Twinkie contain twenty-two teaspoons of sugar. This causes hypoglycemia, and children lose control.

A man brought in his eight-year-old son, for example, and asked for a prescription for Ritalin because the school would not let him return without this medication. I first questioned diet and the possibility of mineral deficiency. When discussing diet and the harmfulness of a heavy sugar load in the morning, the child piped up and said, "I know when I am bad. It's when lunch is supposed to be served at twelve and is not served until twelve thirty." Obviously, this would be when he is the most hypoglycemic. Breakfast served at his school consisted of pancakes and syrup, waffles and syrup, or sugar-frosted flakes and sweet rolls. This diet is almost guaranteed to produce hypoglycemia by lunchtime, but it's great for the promotion of Ritalin and other stimulants. These stimulants hit the same receptor sites as cocaine, and the children begin to like the stimulants.

One of the most damaging things about ADHD is that children are labeled as "bad." Such a self-image, imposed by adults, is very destructive. I made sure that the eight-year-old and his father in the above example realized that the child was not bad and should not be labeled "bad."

We also have mineral depletion in our diet because nitrogen is replaced in the soil, but minerals are not. A deficiency in magnesium alone can produce marked hyperactivity. And we have airborne toxins in the school and in the home that cause profound hyperactivity and loss of concentration. Doris Rapp MD is one of the top experts in the world on this, and she has dramatic video films of before and after exposure to airborne toxins.

Nonetheless, I have seen many hyperactive children whose mothers went to work before they reached age two; and the hyperactivity, plus loss of impulse control, and lower brain volume all point to the working mother and the subsequent return to infant brain as the major cause of the epidemic of ADHD.

<u>Attention deficit disorder (ADD)</u> might have the same age range-of-origin. As with many other disorders, no data has been collected on this regarding infant separation trauma. There also is a high positive correlation between levels of lead and ADD, which is progressive, all the way to coma. This does not exclude separation traumas from the mix. Toxins and other stress factors can contribute to symptom-defining and symptom-precipitating traumas.

With the schizophrenias, psychotic and nonpsychotic depressions, and borderline personality disorders, there is sufficient data to prove the infant separation trauma origin and, in many instances, to show a fivefold increase in the disorder among those traumatized during specific early months.

All factors nonetheless should be reviewed, even if they are relatively insignificant.

Dyslexia

I cautioned one young man about not letting his wife go to work until the baby was three years old. He decided to let her go to work when the child was between one and two. When I saw him ten years later, his son had dyslexia. I reminded him that I cautioned him not to let his wife work prior to the child's third birthday. His reply was, "Oh no, this is dyslexia. It has to do with the wiring in the brain." I wish I knew the age in months when the mother went to work. That would give a clue as to age of origin of that type of dyslexia. This too needs to be surveyed, and simple survey data might allow us to eliminate various types of dyslexia.

Alcohol and Drug Dependence

Alcohol dependence has an early age of origin, but there have been no studies to identify peak age or age range-of-origin. The origin probably relates to prolonged or repeated early stress, such as caused by having an alcohol or drug dependent mother, or one who is severely depressed.

This does not mean that mothers of alcoholics abandoned their babies, and it does not mean that all children of alcoholic mothers become alcoholic. Most often, mothers who imbibe have little awareness of the impact this has on the infant or toddler; and certainly, no harm is intended. They might otherwise be perfect mothers who are attentive to the needs of their children and who would do anything in the world for them. Usually there is no awareness that the baby is being harmed. This is strictly unintentional. Sometimes drinking is planned for after the baby falls asleep, but babies do awaken during the night, and they do recognize a hangover the next day.

The posttraumatic stress disorder mechanism is the same nonetheless. Some report becoming alcoholic with the first drink, while others drink socially for years until one day the stress in the present matches that of the stress in the past and precipitates a return to the earlier time. Often this begins with an important separation in the present, which is coupled with additional stress such as divorce and financial burden. The shift to infancy is called "crossing the invisible line." It is a return to the early feeding situation. The person shifts to the infant-on-the-bottle mind/brain/reality and drinks until the belly is full and passes out. Once the shift is made, recurrences happen with little further provocation. One drink causes the person to return to the infant-on-the-bottle mind/brain/reality.

For many years, I wondered what causes alcoholics, who dread starting an alcoholic binge, to take that first drink, knowing that they might be mugged, robbed, suffer broken bones, and later be hospitalized with terrifying delirium tremens, develop pneumonia, liver failure, ascites, or esophageal varices. I only could picture the infant who is cold, wet, hungry, teething, and crying for minutes and hours—which to the infant seems like days and weeks—until finally someone comes along, picks it up, dries it off, holds it, and feeds it. It must be that moment of bliss that the alcoholic is seeking from the bottle.

Animal studies show that monkeys with early separations from their mothers are more prone to alcoholism. On a large scale, behind the iron curtain of yesteryear, women were paid to stay home the first four months following delivery; but then stipends gradually were reduced until most had to return to work. When the baby reached age two, all mothers were forced to return to work. Reportedly, in some regions, two-thirds became alcoholic.

Drug addictions are similar. In one study, 83 percent of cocaine-addicted patients had mothers who were alcohol or drug addicted. Drug addiction replicates the same infant sequence of putting something in the mouth to feel good.

While great emphasis has been placed on genetic factors, there were no indications of hereditary factors with other primates that were separated early from their mothers and became alcoholic.

It is true that persons in some families are able to tolerate large quantities of alcohol without noticeable effect, and this appears in future generations. But Voyager RNA was discovered at the turn of the twenty-first century, and it provides for a shuffling of the gene sequence until the right combination allows for tolerance of whatever is producing chronic illness. This shuffling of gene sequence is passed on to the next generation, so in that sense, a portion of the tolerance for alcohol can be considered hereditary. It can develop in one generation and then be passed on to the next.

I leave the matter of genetics to the geneticists, but it is clear that early separation trauma produces drug and alcohol dependent offspring.

Idiot Savant and Other Unusual Geniuses

The few that I encountered had suffered early separation traumas too, which caused earlier brain structures to be activated and to develop in unique fashion. Recently an eight-year-old child was brought in who had been placed on huge doses of antipsychotic medication and was showing early signs of liver failure. There had been early separation trauma in the first two years of his life, but I could not pinpoint a specific age in months. The parents just wanted this child to make it through school and adapt to fitting in with society. The medications were a misguided attempt to get him to conform to a very low level of function. Meanwhile, this child had incredible artistic abilities, drawing from sight, at age four, what I might never be able to do. Was this a matter of remaining fixed in a particular early region of brain that had these unique abilities?

Two more incredible mathematical geniuses I met had trauma at fifteen and a half months. Is this the age of development of the angular gyrus, the area of brain that develops for mathematics? These things should be tested. Simple surveys can reveal the answers, very quickly and without huge expenditures.

Eating Disorders

At what age do we worry about what a person puts in the mouth? Or whether the person is eating or not eating? Or whether the person burps up its food? That, of course, is with a baby. It receives lots of attention, with persons plying it with spoonfuls of food and heaping praise for eating and rebuke for not eating.

This is replicated on eating disorders units in mental hospitals across the country. Everything they eat is carefully monitored. They are continuously watched. Essentially, the early feeding process is repeated several times every day, and then they are watched to make sure they do not burp up.

I have seen both anorexia and bulimia reverse with this simple understanding, combined with another primary treatment principle discussed in chapter 14. One schizophrenic patient also had anorexia. She was tall and weighed only eighty-seven pounds during her hospitalization, but when she looked into the mirror, she would think, "My god, I am huge." That obviously was earlier reality because only to a little baby does an eighty-seven-pound woman look enormous. After return to adult mind and brain, her weight returned to normal—without treatment in an eating disorders unit and without any other treatment for anorexia. A simple return to adult reality is all that was required.

Cannibalism: The Strangest of All Eating Disorders

The case of Gary Heidnik, who chained women in his basement because he wanted babies, took an even more bizarre turn when he ground the flesh of the first one who died and began feeding it to the other victims. More strange still was the fact that he placed neatly wrapped body parts in the freezer and labeled them "arm," "thigh," etc. His intention was to feed these to babies as they were being weaned from the breast.

This last detail clarifies origin. Psychoanalyst Bertram Lewin described the infant's oral triad, which is the wish to eat, to be eaten, and to sleep. The baby first sucks on the breast. Then when it begins developing teeth and starts to bite, its wish becomes the wish to devour mother.

As strange as this might seem, it is a common phenomenon but not recognized. Have you ever affectionately said to a toddler, "I'm going to gobble you up" only to get a response of extreme fright? This is because your thought touches that of the baby. And what is the derivation of your own comment?

When the mother is pregnant with a second child, the first can have the desire to be the one who is inside the mother and constantly surrounded by her, receiving her constant attention. This, in part, could contribute to the wish to be eaten. It also might be one origin of claustrophobia. When the baby starts to bite, it can have the wish to devour the mother and have the mother inside at all times.

As a result of analyzing Gary Heidnik (after he was caught), I received calls from all over the world reference other cases of cannibalism. The strangest came from Germany when one man convinced another man to let him eat him. Before finishing the last meal, he began advertising on the Internet for others who wanted to be eaten, offering the opportunity for the next person to dine with him on the remains of the first. Surprisingly enough, there were more than forty persons wishing to be eaten! Why should this be so prevalent? Perhaps this early desire is more universal than we might think.

Section IV

Prevention and Treatment

Three levels of prevention are identified, based on new understanding of mental and emotional disorders.

Primary treatment principles are described. Clinical examples and large-scale studies confirm a powerful dimension of treatment which few even suspect.

Examples are given of spontaneous cures without treatment.

Fifteen treatment modalities are outlined, with special emphasis on meditation, love energy and programmed dreams.

The quality of mothering and the erosion of societal values are examined. These are distinguished from the need to avoid early separation traumas.

Chapter 13

Prevention of Serious Mental and Emotional Disorders

<u>Three Levels of Prevention:</u>
1. Prevention or attenuation of original trauma
2. Prevention or modification of second trauma, which prevents the disorder from ever occurring
3. Prevention of a recurrence among those with a disorder, through new treatment modalities

<u>The first level is prevention of original trauma.</u> The importance of the delayed posttraumatic stress disorder model is that for the first time, it is possible to institute primary prevention.

Schizophrenia can be prevented through the careful identification and elimination or modification of original trauma during the critical stages of development in infancy. Among those infants where trauma cannot be avoided, it at least can be modified, and the infant provided additional assurance and comfort. This is a public health issue that deserves full media attention and then should be taught in schools and to mental health professionals worldwide. Meanwhile, you can counsel your own friends and relatives with regard to the importance of infant separations. Do not let traumatic separations occur. If the child is screaming at the top of its lungs, it is because a separation is too traumatic for it to handle. This must be taken very seriously. If the child screams upon separation at age two or three, this is because it already experienced separation trauma much earlier, and this calls for very careful handling. You must not intensify the trauma at that point.

For the first level of prevention, the mother should stay home with the baby. Do not be led astray by the talk shows that tell how to pick the best babysitter or the best daycare. Recognize the danger in the excuse that the mother has to work. The baby would prefer to live in a cardboard box with the mother than to have a comfortable bed without her. Meanwhile, the father must do everything possible to make the mother feel happy and secure.

When the mother's absence is unavoidable—if she is hospitalized for example—the next best thing might be for a familiar family member to stay in the same home with the baby. Separating from mother and separating from home and everyone the baby knows adds to the trauma. Babies also do not travel well, even with the mother. World travel with the mother can be traumatic because unfamiliar surroundings can distract the mother and be overwhelming to the baby.

If the mother becomes extremely upset about a personal tragedy, it is critically important that she resolve her worries as quickly as possible, focus her attention on the baby, and try to make the baby feel secure.

Recently, a woman was given an independent medical examination by a psychiatrist working for an insurance carrier. She had been assaulted and raped and thought she would be killed a few years earlier while on her job, but she was making good progress in her therapy. During the examination, the psychiatrist reviewed all aspects of the rape and assault, and this rekindled her anxiety and terror associated with the assault.

He then began questioning where she lived, what time her husband left for work each day, when he returned, where her parents lived, and details about her parents. She was from a third world country, was unfamiliar with some of the strange customs in this country, and did not know what to make of the inappropriate questioning. It seemed to her that he wanted to know when her husband was away so that he could harm her, and that he might even want to harm her family.

She began perceiving him as another assailant who was gathering information so he could bring harm to her and her family. When I saw her with the baby several days later, she was crying; and for the first time, the baby was crying. They both continued to cry during subsequent visits. She remained so upset after the inappropriate interview that over the next six months, the baby remained the same weight of seventeen pounds in a classical failure-to-thrive syndrome.

Babies are sensitive to more than just the feelings of the mother. They seem to have an awareness of the thoughts and the perceived dangers of the mother. This would hold true for conscious *and* unconscious thoughts.

My first comments were about the baby crying, whereas it had not cried in the office before. The focus of our visits was to have her give all attention to the baby and make sure the baby was secure and happy. This helped, but the baby still continued to sense her fear. She would have required much more intensive therapy to reduce more of her fear and anxiety because extreme posttraumatic stress disorder had been reactivated, but our time was limited. There now is great concern about this baby's future because such an original trauma will set the stage for the later development of a serious disorder.

In 1999, I was asked by the Turkish Psychological Association to train their members to work in the earthquake disaster area. My first focus was on the babies. Babies are extremely sensitive. On the airplane to Istanbul, the grief was so heavy and palpable that even the babies were crying softly. One of the first things I taught was that if an infant lost its mother, it must have one permanent replacement mother right away. If the mother or the baby were hospitalized, they must be kept in the same room if possible unless the mother's injuries were too severe.

There were 50,000 killed, 50,000 in hospitals, and 200,000 living in tents. I even emphasized on Turkish national TV that it is critical that mothers not focus on having lost their homes or their friends and family members; they must focus on the needs of the baby.

Drug and Alcohol Dependence

Drug- or alcohol-addicted women need to overcome their dependency on abusive substances prior to having children, and they should be in a position to devote their time to the baby. They need to plan so that they do not have to go to work when a baby needs their attention.

Laura Schlessinger, better known as Dr. Laura, is famous for saying that even birds know enough to build a nest first.

Somehow child rearing no longer seems part of everyone's ideal. Last year, I spoke with a nurse who was quite pregnant, and I asked if she was planning to stay home with her baby. "Not me," she replied. "I'm not a stay-at-home mom! My five-year-old gets two hours of my time when I come home, and that's all I can take of him."

Obviously, the five-year-old is traumatized enough by the early separation that he fusses and cries, and the nurse (mother) can't take a fussy child. Also striking is the fact that to this woman, it was something beneath her to be a stay-at-home mom. This is a change in societal values. In some segments of society, it apparently is looked down upon to be a stay-at-home mom. Clearly, there is little understanding or appreciation of the needs of a young child, not to mention the crucial importance of that career called "motherhood."

<u>The second level of prevention</u> is the prevention of an initial psychosis, major depression, or other serious disorder in the vulnerable teenager or young adult. If we prevent the initial episode, we prevent the disorder. We can identify the vulnerable teenager or young adult by knowing the early history of the individual or by recognizing early warning signs or precursors of schizophrenia.

Once we identify the vulnerable child, the next task is to educate that person as to the cause and mechanism of mental illness, discuss any upset feelings they have had, identify these as being associated with separation or rejection, explain the mechanisms, and caution him or her about what precipitates a greater upset. Any separation, rejection, or failure should be closely monitored.

Many teenagers commit suicide because of being rejected by a girlfriend or boyfriend. Teenagers and young adults must be closely monitored for such separation traumas and for any change in behavior, such as suddenly becoming distant.

Separation can cause a flashback to what they experienced as a rejection much earlier in life. To the infant or toddler, the mother is the whole world; and if she is not there, that is the end of the world. Many teenagers feel it is the end of the world when a girlfriend or boyfriend rejects them. This is a shift to an earlier time. This is infant reality. To the adult, there are seven billion people on the planet; and if one leaves, so what! It might be very upsetting, but there are many more choices.

O. Spurgeon English had a unique way of getting the adolescent to recognize this. He would ask, "How many people do you think you will date before you settle down and get married?" Likely, the adolescent will say ten or twenty, at which time they have brought themselves out of the one-year-old reality that the whole world consists of one person.

Again, this is not the mother's fault. Most often it is an unfortunate set of circumstances at a critical stage of development. If you happen to have lost a child, or if you know of someone who has, the deep pain usually can be reduced with the programmed dream. This technique is detailed in chapter 19.

The third level of prevention is the prevention of a recurrence among those who already have the disorder. Based on the new understanding of the disease process, new therapeutic techniques have been developed for this purpose, and these are highly effective.

Chapter 14

The Primary Treatment Principles for Patient and Therapist

<u>The First Treatment Principle</u>

Correct understanding is vitally important for treatment. Once revealed, it is so easy to comprehend that perhaps it should be explained first, whenever clinically feasible. This might take only a very short period of time. Details are added as patient and therapist make important new discoveries along the way. It is like putting together a puzzle that one has struggled with for years without understanding. Knowing the origin and mechanism of one's disorder provides the foundation for further insight. This gives a simple framework within which to explore. Otherwise, treatment is like entering a foreign city without a road map and not knowing the language.

When asked to evaluate the notorious Gary Heidnik—who chained women in his basement because he wanted babies—I notarized a statement on the way to the prison (based on newspaper accounts of his behavior), saying it was my opinion the origin of his disorder was close to eighteen months, and therefore I predicted his brother was that much younger. When we met, I explained the origin and mechanism for his schizophrenia in the first ten minutes and then showed him the notarized statement. He immediately saluted me and shook my hand. Imagine how surprised he was. For twenty-five years, with as many hospitalizations, he had remained completely in the dark, along with his physicians, as to what was wrong with his mind. It is not uncommon to see such great relief, as he expressed, when a lifelong mystery finally is solved.

Regrettably, there are some who might foolishly regard this report as a boast of my unique skills or abilities. Actually, the point being made is that any person of average intelligence can do the same, once the simple origin and mechanism for schizophrenia have been revealed and are understood. I was a month off in my estimate and felt disappointed, but had I met him first, I would have said seventeen months because of an oddity in his behavior and strangeness in his affect not reported in the news.

As I was writing this chapter, a woman called to tell about her forty-seven-year-old son who was in prison. She said he was in prison but that he really did not understand what he was doing was wrong, and she attributed this to dyslexia. As she spoke a few more minutes, I suspected something more serious and asked about younger siblings. His brother was eighteen months younger. I explained this was within the age range-of-origin for schizophrenia, that birth of a sibling was the most frequent single cause in his generation, and some of his symptoms resembled aspects of that disorder. I assured her that his condition was not her fault. Just the birth of a sibling at that age increased the incidence of schizophrenia approximately fivefold. I also let her know what had been holding him back from recovery for the thirty-five years he had been in treatment, and that her plans for him after he was discharged would only keep him in the infirm state. She understood in just a few minutes and was relieved to know. She also clearly understood it was not her fault.

Correct understanding of origin and mechanism enables the patient and family to see what leads to recovery and what makes it worse and why. Then, for the first time, they can direct themselves toward permanent recovery, and they can examine each thought/word/feeling/action and know whether it is helpful or harmful. Without this, they might just remain lost.

Depression, as we have seen, shares a common origin and mechanism with schizophrenia and other serious disorders. Only the age of origin is different. We already reviewed the scientific reasons and proofs for that mechanism, and the findings have been tested and confirmed on large numbers of patients thus far.

We have seen the parallel with war trauma, and we can identify with the horrors of war, but it is hard for us to imagine why a baby would react as strongly to events that do not seem traumatic to us as adults. It is hard for us to imagine because we have forgotten how we thought and what we felt during the first years of life.

It is very important for us to recognize the shift to the earlier time and realize that once the person makes that shift, there exists simultaneously two minds in one skull: the mind and brain of the adult combined with that of the troubled infant.

Understanding this is important because it makes clear the direction to aim for recovery: one must do everything possible to move from infant mind and brain to that of the adult and nothing to cause movement in the opposite direction.

This holds true not only for the psychoses from the first two years of life but for the nonpsychotic depressions from the next year of life. This is because the same mechanism applies.

The classical example for nonpsychotic depression from the last century is Marilyn Monroe. When she was two and a half years old, her mother went to a mental hospital. At that early age, Ms. Monroe would experience this as "Mommy went away and left me," and she would view her mother as a goddess. Consequently, she could only blame herself and hate herself for any disharmony in the relationship. This self-blame would be according to the two-and-a-half-year-old's concept of being "bad," "ugly," or "unlovable." Ms. Monroe's entire life was a desperate attempt to make herself beautiful and lovable; yet in the end, in spite of having won the love and admiration of half the world, she re-experienced her earlier reality of being unlovable once more.

We see these shifts to earlier mind more clearly all the time, and the more we recognize the many variations of the shift in others, the better we can understand the shift in ourselves. It is through correct understanding that we equip ourselves with the tools for making change for moving from the infant/toddler mind back to that of the adult.

The Second Treatment Principle

The second treatment principle is perhaps the most important one of all. It can result in spontaneous cure, without persons understanding or even questioning what caused the change. Symptoms simply disappear, and no one recognizes or understands why. It even appears in large survey data, yet still no one sees or comprehends.

To understand this blindness requires realizing that we cannot have divided interests. We cannot mingle our desire to help others heal, with the desire to receive a research grant, or to publish a paper, or to find a drug that can be sold for profit, or to win popularity, or to find answers that others will accept, or to avoid criticism by endorsing the status quo. Even if the men and women conducting the studies are sincere and filled with integrity, they cannot do their best work for a company that only seeks profits, or for an institution that is motivated primarily by research grants. Such influences affect all who participate.

We must focus exclusively on the patient and family, what caused the problem and how to correct it. This is a challenge, for it is a narrow path that leads to truth, and we are easily sidetracked along the way.

This second treatment principle is the most critical factor for rapid permanent recovery. Yet it is not what people want to hear. It might be what they, most of all, do *not* want to hear. It involves extreme sensitivities and stirs strong emotional reaction in laypersons and professionals alike.

Nonetheless, it is the one factor that alone can result in spontaneous cure, even without any treatment whatsoever.

For this reason, this main treatment modality is presented only after providing a thorough understanding of origin and mechanism. Without such preliminary understanding, the reader might dismiss everything and never benefit from findings that can move a person beyond a serious mental or emotional disorder and might never learn how to prevent the same from occurring in future generations.

This major treatment principle involves change in one's environment. It is not too different from the recommendations of Alcoholics Anonymous. In AA, persons are taught to avoid "people, places, and things" that cause them to move back into their addiction. Recovery, in fact, is predicated upon total abstinence from the abusive substance. No matter how much one knows about the disorder, total abstinence is required for recovery. It is recognized as being pivotal to recovery. This important treatment principle is equally pivotal for recovery from schizophrenia, but few recognize it. Few have even noticed. But the reaction to the concept is very strong. It is every bit as strong as was the reaction to infantile sexuality at the turn of the nineteenth century. That concept is accepted now as fact among professionals and laypersons alike. So we have something pivotal, something that is key for recovery, yet something—like infantile sexuality—which not only had gone undetected but which, when revealed, is met with extreme emotional reaction and extreme psychological resistance.

To develop our thinking further, let us first consider how we sometimes behave differently in relation to specific people. We behave one way to relatives and family members, another way to strangers, and still other ways to friends of the same gender versus friends of the opposite sex. We differ in our relationships with clergy versus law enforcement versus children. We take on different mind-sets, different roles, and we behave differently in relation to different people and different categories of people. This you understand. We become a parent when we see a child in trouble; we become a polite model citizen when we encounter a police officer; sometimes we take on a holy air when we encounter clergy; we are aggressive adversaries in relation to others on the football field, etc. This is not to say we are phonies, but we do become different people in different situations. Christians will recall the apostle Paul saying he became all things to all people. This is an automatic blending-in process and nearly everyone does it.

Now the question is, do people become schizophrenic or depressed in relation to certain people? The answer is, yes—a resounding yes! Once a mental disorder has been precipitated or once a psychotic or depressive process has been activated, it becomes reactivated in relation to certain individuals. Remember how we define schizophrenia? It is the coexistence of the mind/brain/reality/feelings/behavior of the adult and the awakened mind/brain/reality/feelings/behavior of the infant. Depression, likewise, is the coexistence of the mind/brain/reality/feelings/behavior of the adult, combined with that of the two-to-three-year-old.

Thus, if the patient has an infant-to-adult relationship with another person, any contact with that other person will cause a shift to the earlier mind/brain/

reality/feelings and behavior—i.e., a shift into the depths of their illness. Regardless how much another person might want to help, the nature of the relationship itself can destroy all chances of permanent recovery.

This is like the relationship between an alcoholic and the bottle. It might be a very fine bottle of wine, treasured by connoisseurs; but one sip takes the alcoholic back to the infant-on-the-bottle mind/brain/reality, and he drinks until the belly is full and he passes out. This is the same mechanism with schizophrenia and depression.

Just as the substance can be the finest in the world, so the person in relation to whom we shift to the earlier age can be the finest in the world, but the reality of the shift in relation to that person remains. And other people shift in relation to us. If we shift to infant or toddler reality, then nearly everyone relates to us as though we were infants or toddlers.

This becomes particularly clear in mental hospitals, yet few recognize it: the hospital staff gives patients crayons and coloring books and speaks baby talk to them. This is one more example of how persons relate to one another. The mental health team relates to the patient as a parent does to an infant, and often to a naughty one at that. This is counterproductive. It keeps the patients locked into earlier mind and brain. The patients themselves need to recognize this and not permit it.

Still, we have not arrived at the primary treatment recommendation. It has to do with the delayed posttraumatic stress disorder mechanism and the return to the original symptom-defining trauma. Once that trauma is activated in the combat veteran, even popcorn popping in the next room can be mistaken for machine-gun fire in the distance and can cause the veteran to experience the reality that he is back in war.

Similarly with schizophrenia, once the infant mind has been awakened, it takes very little to reawaken. Thus it is crucial for patient, family, and therapist to recognize what it is that causes a return to the original trauma and what is it that keeps the infant mind and brain active.

Nearly everything you have heard or read or know will disagree with this primary treatment recommendation; yet I have not met anyone, even those who most vehemently oppose it, who has ever tried it or has direct knowledge of the result.

In understanding this, first we must realize that the original traumatic event, as experienced by the infant or toddler, was an unrecognized fear of separation; and we must realize that the infant or toddler at that time—particularly if separation involved the death of a parent—desperately sought the parent or any other family member in much the same way a drowning victim struggles to grasp a floating object. If you understand this, then you understand that once *that* particular part of the infant mind and brain has been activated and a first psychotic or major depressive episode has occurred, *any contact with an original nuclear family member can keep the infant portion of the mind and brain active and in high gear*. This—more than any other factor—serves to perpetuate the disorder.

"Oh no, that's not so," you might be thinking. I'm sorry, but I truly believe it is and will back my conviction with evidence that it is so—particularly, if the encounter occurs prior to a lengthy period of separation, growth, and independence. My experience has convinced me that all a parent or any original nuclear family member has to do is have a brief encounter with someone whose infant mind previously was activated, and the infant mind can become *re*activated once more.

This is because of the infant's intense needs for that family member. It literally can spring forth, become active, and take over. Then the earlier regions of brain, which become reactivated as a result, increase production of their neurotransmitters; and the higher cortical structures that developed later become correspondingly less active and undergo disuse atrophy. And as a result, we have a neurobiological disorder.

This is a horrible fate for anyone to experience because the parent is the one person who would do anything in the world to help the child, yet the more the parent does and the harder the parent tries, the more entrenched and permanent the condition can become.

More traditional treatment approaches might bring small gains in an unending battle, and these small gains foster hope. These are taken as signs that what one is doing is helpful, but in my broad experience, the gains are small indeed compared to the gains made through total separation. There is no comparison. With correct understanding and a complete, total separation from all original nuclear family members, disorders of recent onset can simply disappear, even without further intervention; and long-standing conditions can stabilize and begin to improve.

There are a few noted psychoanalysts who are able to analyze schizophrenia successfully while the patient remains in contact with family, but the burden of treatment might be lighter if they analyzed the patient when there is no contact with original family. Psychoanalysts are reluctant and usually refuse to analyze a patient who is alcoholic and continues to drink, or who is drug addicted and continues to take drugs. This is very similar, only instead of a toxic substance it is a toxic relationship.

Separation is not unnatural and is not without benefit in other recognized realms of the maturation process. It is commonly accepted that teenagers, who separate and go away to college, suddenly begin to mature at an accelerated pace. This is because at home, they are children in relation to parents and tend to remain as children. Separation helps them grow. It is part of their maturation process. This is all part of the same continuum. Thus, when persons shift to reality/feelings/behavior of the first years of life, separation is a natural way to help bring them out.

After psychosis first occurs, there are two minds in one skull: the adult mind and the awakened mind of the infant. If there is a box of candy in a room and an adult and a child are present, it is the child who clamors for the candy. Likewise, if there is an adult and an awakened infant mind in the same skull, and a family member is present, it is the infant mind that comes to the forefront. Sometimes, the more the parent does and the harder the parent tries, the worse the condition becomes. The effort a family exerts to help a psychotic child might be sufficient to cure an army of neurotics, but the condition only worsens. It is like struggling in quicksand. A complete separation and disassociation between patient and family early in the course of the illness—along with just an hour or two of correct understanding—easily would eliminate a very large portion of all schizophrenia.

This does not mean abandoning the patient. Carefully structured support and help at a distance, through other people in a therapeutically structured environment, is a key to rapid and permanent recovery. Within the first few months of total separation, medications often must be eliminated because they become too sedating.

The Trap of Schizophrenia

Once the infant mind is activated, the patient is an infant in relation to the parent, and no infant will let go of the parent. This is a trap from *both* directions: from the other direction, no parent will give up a baby. Both cling with tenacity. Sometimes one clings more than the other. Special effort must be made to get patient and family to understand this trap and to learn how to escape from it. Otherwise, the patient can remain caught in an endless cycle of psychosis, hospitalization, recovery, returning home to family, and recurrent psychosis. No one would treat alcoholism by prescribing vodka, yet the majority of mental health professionals try to treat schizophrenia while maintaining a relationship between patient and family. Consequently, most therapists believe that it is not possible to cure; and they look to diminish symptoms and frequency of recurrent episodes through medication, never realizing that with an adequate period of separation—combined with psychotherapy, growth, development, and independence—there is a strong probability that the condition will not recur.

Patient and family must be encouraged to try a complete separation—without even a telephone call—for at least a month; and if there is progress, they should continue it for another month and another month. The level of recovery must be communicated only through the therapist or some other intermediary because one telephone call per month can erase any gain and perpetuate the disorder. After the third month, there usually is substantial gain and noteworthy change has occurred. Medicines have to be reduced by half or eliminated altogether. This is because the reactivated infant part of the brain is frightened and produces more of the neurotransmitters involved in the disease process, but as the person moves away from the infant mind and brain, back into the adult mind and brain, the unconscious fear experienced in earlier mind and brain begins to disappear. It is the unspoken terror of separation that requires sedation with a major tranquilizer. Even the adult mind would remain alert after taking a major tranquilizer if it were experiencing a similar overwhelming and imminent threat to survival. When there is no contact with family, the infant mind is deactivated along with its unconscious threat, and then any powerful medication becomes far too sedating.

When separation is structured in a therapeutic way, with help at a distance set in place, it is an act of unselfish love—and one that ultimately is rewarded. Separation does not mean abandonment of the patient. It is a carefully structured separation with support at a distance built into the plan, and it must occur with agreement. It cannot be an angry, rejecting separation such as saying, "Get out. I never want to see you again." That would precipitate an immediate shift into infancy. Instead it should be, "We really care and we want the very best for you. The doctor says this will put your life back on track so let's give it a try."

With separation alone, many delusional systems, in excess of ten years, simply disappear—even without treatment or understanding. Methods for implementing the separation will be described in later chapters.

Early Clinical Examples of the Effect of Contact

In the late 1960s and early 1970s, after training and at the very beginning of private practice, a number of clinical examples occurred in close sequence that were so extraordinary I never will forget. The intensity and frequency of the early cases, in retrospect, seem to defy the likelihood of occurring by chance alone.

One of the first among the early cluster of striking examples was a young lady who was very psychotic. It took several weeks on a locked ward in the hospital to achieve sufficient recovery to transfer her to an open unit. The family had not been allowed to visit because they upset her.

Shortly after being transferred to the open unit, her parents visited; and within minutes, she became acutely psychotic. She was screaming, delusional, and wanted to die. She immediately had to be transferred back to the locked unit. Again she recovered and went to the open unit, and again the parents visited, and again she became acutely psychotic. This same scenario was repeated five more times over the next fourteen weeks. It was most striking. She would recover from the delusions, transfer to the open ward, parents would visit or call on the telephone, and immediately she would become psychotic. After a total of twelve transfers, the family saw the connection and agreed to separate. Never again did she require hospitalization or medication or psychotherapy. She became independent, worked, eventually married, had several children and, as of last count, five grandchildren. After several years of solid stabilization, she was able to resume limited contact with family without the shift back into infant mind/brain/reality/feelings and behavior.

The suddenness of the many shifts into insanity, and the numerous transfers from ward to ward, were so striking that they demanded careful scrutiny of this phenomenon in the future; yet in spite of the dramatic changes, no one at the hospital made special note of this in any way. No one thought to apply the principle to the next patient. To me, the nonresponse by trained professionals was as striking as the many sudden recurrent psychotic episodes!

Variations of this same phenomenon repeat throughout this book and have been noted throughout the ages. Ezekiel wrote about those who have eyes to see but do not see, ears to hear but do not hear. Jeremiah and Isaiah describe the same, and this is repeated several times in the New Testament. I mention this here because of the number of simple observations made, from cover to cover of this book, which seem clear and obvious, but for some reason have not been noticed—and when pointed out, they have been ignored!

Back to the clinical vignettes: another lady, who graduated from a teachers college shortly before her first psychotic episode, had been hospitalized each year for ten years before I was asked to treat her in the hospital. The first part of the treatment involved total separation from family. The separation, combined with just a little understanding, enabled her to recover well enough that she never required hospitalization again. One day, however, friends took her to the synagogue for a funeral service for a relative. She was perfectly normal during the ride with friends, but then her mother walked in and sat next to her. Immediately, she jumped up and began screaming and batting away hallucinatory objects as she stormed out of the synagogue. I felt deep sorrow for the pain this caused her mother, but after that experience, her mother recognized what I had been describing and decided to adhere to the total separation. The daughter recovered quickly and remained well. Her mother was very grateful for her recovery, and her daughter had no more psychotic episodes over the next fifteen years. Gradually limited contact became possible.

Following the mother's death, the patient recovered still further and found employment as a full-time schoolteacher with the Philadelphia public school system for several years. She still had a few oddities about her behavior after the many years of psychosis, but she functioned relatively well. After seven years of employment, the school system fired her, which precipitated an upset, but she did not require hospitalization. Another physician placed her on Risperdal, even though she had not required medication since the time I first treated her more than fifteen years earlier. One dramatic change was evident, which also was observed by her best friend. The medication took the "spark" out of her. She always had been lively and energetic, even though marked with idiosyncrasy, but with the medicine, it was as if she had lost her soul.

Another schoolteacher from New Jersey was married, had been away from her family for many years, and was leading a relatively normal life. Then one summer, she visited her parents in the South; and when she returned, she was like a zombie. She wore a frozen expression and was numb. During infancy, needs are very great; and if the needs are not met, this can be so overwhelming that the infant becomes numb as a means of coping with the pain. The infant simply shuts off all feelings and emotions, and that is exactly what this patient had done. The symptom of numbness identifies her trauma as occurring prior to eighteen months.

Another example is a young man who was so suicidal and depressed that he just wanted to die. His entire depression disappeared in the hospital within one day of my explaining the origin and mechanism for his depression and separating him from family. The separation was complete, without even a telephone call. He quickly was able to return to school and had no traces of his depression.

Then during football practice, he injured his ankle and had to wear a cast for a while. A couple of weeks later, his mother—who still lived in the vicinity—spotted him from across a parking lot, waved to him, and just pointed to his cast as if to say "what happened to you?" There was no verbal communication, just her pointing and noting there was *something wrong* with his foot. This remote inference to something wrong with him immediately plummeted him into severe suicidal depression once more, and he had to be hospitalized the very next day.

More examples will be given later, but it is noteworthy that striking examples such as these went practically unnoticed by the psychiatric community. Why should this be so? Such examples surely did not occur only in one practice.

What is it that blinds the eyes of the viewer? Why are such obvious things overlooked?

Hidden Confirmation in Large Research Studies

This blindness holds true for large research studies as well where persons are looking right at the cause and do not see it.

In the largest study of its kind, G.W. Brown of London was commissioned by the Medical Research Council of England to conduct a study of what factors in the post-mental hospital environment lead to rehospitalization. In 1966, he reported a survey on 339 post-mental hospital patients. One factor alone stood out, and this was not whether they took medicine or not. It was whether they went home or went anywhere else to live. Those who went home returned to the mental hospital.

This was an unacceptable finding. It must not be so. Family members are the ones who care the most. It must be something else. That finding was arbitrarily rejected.

The unacceptable finding led to an intense search for what else might explain it. This search *did* lead to important observations that are helpful, but they do not go far enough. They discovered a positive correlation between recurrent illness and the amount of *expressed emotion* in the family, which they quickly labeled the *EE factor*. Indeed, it is now well established that recurrent illnesses are fewer if there is less expressed emotion (EE factor) in family.

This certainly is an improvement and definitely should be utilized whenever family therapy is used for schizophrenia and other psychoses.

Far more effective than reducing the EE factor, however, is eliminating it altogether. A *zero* EE factor, achieved through a total separation and disassociation from original nuclear family, is immeasurably better. It is the same difference as an alcoholic who decides to abstain instead of merely reducing alcohol intake.

Recall the lad whose mother spotted him from across the parking lot and pointed to his broken foot? That's all the EE factor he needed to plummet back into suicidal depression. And the woman whose mother sat down alongside her in the synagogue? Sometimes that is all the EE factor it takes.

What was missed in the EE factor research is the understanding that contact returns the person to the first years of life when the infant/toddler experienced what *it* considered to be a threat of abandonment. The greater the expressed emotion, the more the contact represents an overwhelming threat of separation to the infant mind.

The EE factor studies were important in that they revealed a correlation between expressed emotion and recurrent illness, and they also revealed the effect of rejection, which is critical in the understanding of mental and emotional disorders. When the patient is not fully recovered, even helpful suggestions come across as criticism and rejection. Screaming things at the patient only causes the patient to sink faster into psychosis. The two things to avoid, prior to full and permanent recovery, are (1) original nuclear family, because this reactivates the infant part of the mind and (2) rejection or failure, because the infant interpreted early circumstances to mean a threat of rejection or separation.

Another large-scale study was conducted by the Ukrainian National Academy of Science. I had just explained my findings to a division head there, and he started to chuckle. One of his researchers hypothesized that there was less schizophrenia in Switzerland because they lived at a higher elevation, which could increase the production of the body's natural endorphins in the brain, and this might lower the incidence of schizophrenia. So they took a group of schizophrenics to the top of a mountain, and after a few months, they were symptom free. Then they returned from the mountain, and after a few months, all were symptomatic again. The division head understood my explanation and immediately recognized what caused the recovery to come and go.

Brief Examples of Dramatic Recoveries without Treatment

One lady described having schizophrenia for fifteen years—except for the two years when she lived in Spain with relatives she had never met. It is difficult to understand why she did not return to Spain to live, except for "the trap of schizophrenia" and the strong pull from both directions. Many prefer to maintain contact with original family and continue to suffer with schizophrenia. I always give the patient this option, but I encourage patient and family to first try a month of separation, and then add a month and another month without contact, so they can see for themselves the dramatic changes that occur.

One of the most humble persons I have known is Dr. John Nash of *A Beautiful Mind* fame. His degree of warmth is a reflection of what he must have received from his parents early in life. Based on the movie, I predicted there was a separation trauma just beyond age fifteen months. Later, I learned that when he was fifteen months old, the stock market was 400, and when he was sixteen months old in October 1929, it was 200. Many lost everything practically overnight. Mothers, who had focused all attention on their babies, suddenly were concerned about losing their homes or having enough food to feed the family. This trauma, related to the 1929 market crash, produced an emotional separation trauma that I had described many years earlier in the textbook *Delayed Posttraumatic Stress Disorders from Infancy*. The age at time of trauma provides the common denominator for symptoms—and unique child-rearing practices, combined with quality of mothering, accounts for symptom variation.

The last time I met with Dr. Nash, I told him, without hesitation, when his symptoms would have disappeared. I said, "Your symptoms would have disappeared after your last parent died." He replied that his father died in the 1950s, his mother in 1969, and his last hospitalization—and last medication for that matter—was in 1970. I then learned that he moved in with his sister after his mother died, which accounts for the last hospitalization. Spontaneous recovery usually requires separation from *all* nuclear family members.

The prediction was an easy determination to make because I have never seen such a severe and lengthy illness go into that degree of spontaneous remission without a period of total separation from original nuclear family. He did not return to live with his sister.

At times, one family member will have more impact on the patient than another. This does not mean that the person is doing something wrong. It means that the relationship is more prone to shifting to parent-infant.

One man we met on a family vacation in Boqueron Bay, Puerto Rico, said a physician at a VA hospital told him he had schizophrenia and would have to take Thorazine for the rest of his life. This man showed no signs of the illness whatsoever. Instead of taking Thorazine, he bought a sailboat and just traveled through South America and the islands for a year with his lady friend, and all symptoms disappeared. We visited for a little while, and he understood right away when I explained the origin and mechanism of his disorder and why his symptoms disappeared.

<u>More Examples of Impact of Family on Patient (Including Successful Treatments that Failed after Patient Reunited with Family)</u>
An eighteen-year-old girl was hospitalized for an acute psychosis. Another psychiatrist told her parents that she had schizophrenia, would never finish high school, and had to take medication for the rest of her life. Contact with parents, while in the hospital, upset her very much; so all visits and phone calls were discontinued. When she recovered from the acute illness, she was sent directly to a commune and had no contact whatsoever with family. In fact, family did not even know where she was living. At the commune, she required no medication; and within three months, she passed her high school equivalency (GED) exam.

After flourishing for more than six months in the new environment and going to work every day, this eighteen-year-old girl made one phone call home to family. It was like an alcoholic taking a drink after six months of sobriety and never again attaining sobriety. I heard from her twenty years later, and she had remained in the trap of schizophrenia. Permanent recovery would have required much more time and further movement in the direction of independence.

A thirty-year-old man with schizophrenia came for treatment. History revealed that he was unable to find employment because of his psychosis, so he turned to crime. He was caught and given a prison sentence. With the separation from family while in prison, he recovered quickly, but when eventually he was released from prison he returned home to live; and there he became acutely psychotic once more.

This whole sequence repeated several times. When he was well, he was highly motivated and even earned a four-year college degree while in prison; but each time he was released, he returned home, became psychotic, could not find employment, and returned to crime.

When finally he came for treatment, he quickly understood the origin and mechanism for his illness and why it kept recurring. The pattern was unmistakable once revealed. We tried to get Social Security for him so he could live independently long enough to find work. It was denied, and he is back in prison once more.

A twenty-year-old man with schizophrenia lived semi-independently after beginning treatment. Contact with family became minimal when they saw the impact that family contact had on him. Still there were occasional telephone calls that always resulted in partial shifts to infancy. At these times, he required a very small dose of medication for a week or two. We met weekly for lunch at a local pub, and he even found a job at a local florist shop. I gave him an old car to provide a greater sense of independence.

Then his mother learned of a treatment center with supervised housing and nurses and social workers to look in on him on a regular basis. There were no restrictions in regard to family contact, and the treatment center was coupled with an outpatient clinic where he received psychotherapy, and both were coupled with a hospital. The arrangement was tight. The center would send patients to the hospital, the hospital to the clinic, and the clinic to the treatment center and vice versa. Nonetheless, in spite of all the potential for good care, his condition deteriorated dramatically.

Massive doses of at least fourteen different antipsychotic, antidepressant, and antiseizure medications were tried, and usually three or four at a time. He even was given a combination of Clozaril and Tegretol—both of which cause agranulocytosis. When these were combined, the expected occurred. Three times in the next three years he was sent for a month to the hospital (insurance covered one month per year). It has been another fifteen years, with more hospitalizations and more new medications. He is but a shadow of what he might have been. Instead of independence, he was protected and kept in close contact, never again advancing toward full recovery.

One forty-year-old journalist, who was hospitalized several times for recurring psychotic episodes, made a permanent separation and became very successful working 300 miles away from her last living relative, her mother. She had a young son whom she was raising, and her trips to the mental hospital interfered with employment and with care for her son. Seven years after moving away, she called to say that her mother died, but she still was appreciative for what the separation did for the both of them and for her son. She had no more psychotic episodes and did not require treatment or medication since making the separation. In going through her mother's belongings, she saw that her mother had joined senior citizen groups and led a much fuller life. Her mother had been caught in the trap too, and with the separation, she too was able to live a life of her own.

Another case was a twenty-five-year-old woman hospitalized for a schizoaffective psychosis with extreme depression and inability to function. Previously, she had numerous hospitalizations for several years under the care of other physicians and never became functional or independent. I insisted upon the total separation, and once she achieved it, she no longer had psychotic depression. She was able to function and live on her own. She had her own apartment, was successful in real estate business, and was thriving. Nearly a year had elapsed and Christmas was approaching. I was pleased with her recovery and thought that maybe we should try a one-hour visit with her mother on Christmas Day. I reasoned that if she regressed, we could just start over with total separation once more.

In retrospect, this made as much sense as an alcoholic celebrating one year of sobriety with a bottle of champagne. The contact caused her to shift back into the infant mind. She cried, could not function, and had the same extreme self-hatred and self-blame as prior to her recovery. Treatment was interrupted, and she never again was able to separate or return to her former level of recovery.

For years after her unfortunate outcome, when people asked how long the total separation should be maintained, the reply was "For as long as the alcoholic must separate from the bottle" because this is a parallel process.

There *are* two minds in one skull, and each wants to survive. Whichever one dominates, it has a strong desire to remain in control and fights for that control. Each has a separate set of realities, feelings, behaviors, likes, and dislikes. Regardless how miserable the infant is, it does not want to relinquish its existence. The line between this and what some describe as possession is very thin. The descriptions have parallel features, and both exhibit self-destructive tendencies. If there is a spirit world, then it is unscientific to disregard this as a possibility in some cases. I have identified the infant mind and the mechanism for shifting back to it. I leave it to theologians to determine matters of possession.

In the mid-1970s, many psychiatrists were questioning what happens to schizophrenia after age fifty because very few were seen in private practice. I wrote in the *Medical Tribune* that this makes sense when we consider the impact of family on patient and realize that not many people have parents after age fifty.

A Sudden Change in Treatment Plan

The recommendation of total, permanent separation ended abruptly one morning when I was awakened again by the same authoritative voice that kept me from getting sidetracked in the stock market twenty years earlier. I still don't know the source of that voice, but I do know "by the fruit" that it is totally good. Each time, it came at the speed of thought, and there was not one extra word. This is an interesting phenomenon and warrants exploration. Thought transference has no language barrier and possibly also has no extra words.

Both times, there was no question about the correctness of the instruction given. This time, the message again was clear and immediately made sense. It provided a better plan. It modified the recommendation of permanent separation. That instruction is indelibly etched in my mind and brain, but since it came at the speed of thought, I can only paraphrase what I was told. The overall content and thrust are accurate nonetheless.

For thirty-nine years, I have programmed dreams and have taught others to obtain enlightened information during the night in the same way. The programmed dreams are amazing, but mine are no more remarkable than those of my patients. This, however, was not like a programmed dream. I had not been thinking about the recommendation of separation from family and had not formulated any question. That powerful voice seemed to be from a different source. It came of its own volition, without my asking. It was intent upon giving a specific instruction, which made total sense and immediately altered my course of treatment.

This message began with: "Four stages of separation:"

1. "Separate because it works."

2. "Allow time for growth, development, independence." [Time for the person to find employment, become independent, develop social relationships, and establish a residence and a circle of friends—in essence, become so solidly fixed in adult mind/brain/reality that it is like a freight train set so firmly back on track that it takes an extraordinary event to derail once more.]
3. "Educate patient and family as to what to do and what to avoid with renewed contact." [This is where the expressed emotion (EE) factor becomes important so that interactions with family, which could cause a return to the infant mind/brain/reality, are minimized.]
4. "Begin [contact] gradually, with a five-minute telephone call between patient and family, followed by careful monitoring of the patient over the next 72 hours." There was a further telepathic impression that the patient should never return home to live with original family.

I noted the confirmation of my original treatment plan in step number 1 because nothing causes more rapid recovery. The second step—which allows time for growth, development, and independence—makes complete sense. This is the direction we aim in treatment, from infant to adult.

The length of time required for this separation will vary from person to person. Several factors come into play: the duration of illness, the severity of the affliction, the amount of criticism expressed (even helpful suggestions can be taken as rejection), the degree of independence achieved, and the degree of stability attained.

The third step is vital, and this is where the findings related to the EE factor are most helpful. Family and patient both must be well aware of what to expect, what to do, and what to avoid. Patient and family need to understand thoroughly the origin and mechanisms of psychosis and depression; both need to know that it is no one's fault. No one is to blame. Usually it is caused by an unfortunate set of circumstances during a critical stage of development, and no one realized the harm it could cause—not even the experts. There must be a mutual sense of understanding and cooperation as well as total forgiveness for mistakes made by either.

Programmed dreams and prayer are important at this stage. They can provide deep insight and revelation into how to relate. This is a learning process. When even one family member programs a dream as to what to do about the relationship, that dream can reach beyond the dreamer, as you will see in the chapter on programmed dreams. It can reach beyond the dreamer and pave the way for a positive result.

It is difficult to determine when to begin the fourth stage of separation, the gradual reuniting of patient with family. This too might be handled best with enlightenment techniques through prayer, meditation, and programmed dreams in addition to clinical judgment. Certainly, the fourth stage must follow careful education of patient and family as to what to do and what to avoid. This educational process with family was not done in earlier cases, at least not to the extent that was needed. Without educating the family, the one-year separation was grossly insufficient for the woman mentioned above who visited her mother for one hour on Christmas Day.

Another patient had trouble even after seven years. She made a full recovery from schizophrenia and anorexia while in the hospital. She adhered strictly to the mandate of no contact with original family because she wanted to be able to rear her infant daughter. The strict separation enabled her eventually to return to a high-level position with a major pharmaceutical company; but once each year, for seven years, she made one phone call home—and each time, she started hearing voices again and required medication for a little while. Proper preparation of patient and family for the renewed contact likely would have made earlier contact possible.

This patient became concerned about another woman at work who had severe anorexia, and she asked the lady if she were having a health problem. The woman replied that she was dying, so my patient told her what she did that eliminated her own anorexia. The woman made the separation, and her anorexia quickly disappeared.

In determining when to try limited contact, it is better to err in the direction of stability rather than allow the infant to take over and never let go again. Some patients do well after only a couple of years of separation. Others require much longer.

<u>Another Example of Renewed Contact without Prior Education of Family</u>
One young lady who had been hospitalized many times tried separating from family at least a dozen times; but after only a short interval, either she or one of her family members would initiate contact, and this

precipitated an immediate psychosis each time. Interestingly enough, she always returned to the same brain cells, the very same thoughts. She would begin screaming that her brothers beat her and her parents went to Israel. This was like a broken record. The brothers merely had tried to restrain her one time when she was psychotic, and she was an adult when her parents traveled to the Middle East. But to her infant mind, these were huge rejections that her infant mind never could forgive. This was a loving family and everyone wanted to help her, but she couldn't remain separate long enough to attain the degree of health required for permanent recovery.

It is very difficult to know what the infant is experiencing, even when it is experiencing extreme threat to its survival. We only become aware of the original level of distress many years later when the patient re-experiences the event as a full-grown adult. Then we can see what the infant was experiencing.

Subtle Signs of Regression

The dramatic shift to florid psychosis, after a period of separation, is easily seen upon renewed contact with original nuclear family; yet few ever recognize the impact that contact with family has. Partly this is because contact is so frequent that change cannot be detected. One brief hello on the telephone sometimes can perpetuate the disorder for months, and contact usually is daily or weekly. This does not allow for sufficient recovery time to enable patient, family, or therapist to recognize the sudden change that occurs with renewed contact.

With correct understanding, combined with total separation and disassociation from original family for three months, most achieve such dramatic recovery that they cannot take medication; or the medicine has to be reduced by half. The overwhelming threat is what the infant was experiencing, and when the person returns to the adult mind, the threat is gone and the medication becomes far too sedating. Contact *following* several months of recovery more likely will produce the dramatic reversals described above, but few ever see this because contact is too frequent.

There are many other reasons why contact with original family is not recognized as the cause of the dramatic shifts that follow, some of which were already discussed:

1. It seems counterintuitive.
2. It flies in the face of long-held norms.
3. Emotional reaction to it is the same as to recommending a separation between mother and baby.
4. People see this as blaming the parent and fear disapproval.
5. It interferes with needs of institutions.
6. Professionals fear public outcry.
7. And last but not least, commercial ventures might suffer loss.

All these factors that lead to the blindness are things that pertain to our needs and desires and have little or nothing to do with love.

While even the dramatic overt signs of regression into psychosis seldom are recognized as relating to contact, the more subtle signs almost never are recognized and acknowledged as relating to contact.

Nonetheless, when there has been a period of separation accompanied by a degree of recovery, it is vitally important to recognize even the most subtle signs of a shift back into the infant mind and brain. Any sign of slipping into earlier mind/brain/reality must be taken seriously because one falling stone can start a landslide. The infant mind has enormous needs, and when these begin to surface, they can erupt like a volcano.

<u>Examples of Subtle Shifts to Infant Mind and Brain</u>

One young man, who was well into recovery from a serious psychosis, made a brief phone call to his family on a Friday. The following Monday, he did not go to work because he had a cold. Ordinarily, this might be an acceptable excuse; but for the previous one and a half years of recovery, he had never missed work. Thus the missing work was a very subtle sign of regression following contact. Babies do not get out of bed to go to work. Even such a subtle sign should not be overlooked.

A twenty-nine-year-old woman who was treated three times a week after hospitalization for depression made a clicking sound with tongue against palate. She thought it was because her sinuses were draining, but it occurred only on Mondays and not on Wednesdays or Fridays. After further exploration, it was learned that on Sundays she had dinner with her mother. The symptom was a partial return to the infant on the breast. Part of her mind actually was back in the early feeding situation, and she always was more upset on these occasions.

A less fortunate example is a man who had been hospitalized every year for the previous eight or ten years with manic psychosis. Treatment started during his last hospitalization. With separation from original family, he made rapid improvement and was discharged to live in a halfway house. Soon he found employment in a local courthouse, and then he moved into an apartment and bought a car. He had not required medication for approximately one and a half years, and there were no signs of psychosis. Then one day he called and said, "Hey, Doc, put me back in the hospital. I changed jobs, and I just can't take the pressure of this new job anymore." I was puzzled and said, "No, something is wrong here. The pressure of a new job should not cause this much problem to you. It must be contact with family again." Then he revealed he had dinner with his mother the night before. It was the first time in several months. On three other occasions, this had happened over the previous year and a half; and each time, it precipitated a recurrence of subtle signs of psychosis, but he had not asked to be rehospitalized.

This is an example of how quickly an avalanche can follow the first rumble. It is difficult to determine which subtle sign will lead back into psychosis. This is why careful education of patient and family prior to contact is so important, and it is why all initial contacts with family must be carefully monitored.

In retrospect, I should have hospitalized him when he asked because soon he was fully back into psychosis, and he never achieved separation again. He began seeing another psychiatrist who told him he had manic psychosis and would need to take medication for the rest of his life. His new psychiatrist was a renowned authority on bipolar disorder, thoroughly versed on what is known in the field; yet in spite of this, the patient was never able to achieve sufficient recovery to hold a menial job.

This example illustrates how even a most esteemed leader in the field, can literally destroy another human being. Simply caring enough about the patient should have inspired a more creative course of treatment that would have prevented this patient's demise. That which is highly esteemed among men really *can* be an abomination instead.

Several years later, this patient returned to visit. He had gained a hundred pounds, looked disheveled, and his sensorium was dull. He had remained on massive doses of medication, which kept him out of the hospital; but he was a mere shadow of the bright, alert, intelligent, and functioning man who was well and held a responsible job in the courthouse during our brief two years of treatment—all without medication and without family contact. The pull of the family was too great once it was re-established. The separation in his case should have been much longer, and there needed to be education of family.

One of the most interesting examples I have seen of a person shifting to the infant reality upon contact with a parent occurred in a thirty-year-old woman I treated for an acute psychosis. She recovered from a paranoid condition during her brief hospitalization. She quickly learned and understood the mechanisms of the mind, and she followed my advice religiously. Her recovery lasted two and one-half years. She had a baby, and she and her husband and child were getting along well. This was many years ago. Earlier that year, she described her husband to me in glowing terms—he was warm, loving, kind, generous, a wonderful husband and a perfect father to the child. Then she noted that she had not seen her parents for a long time, and her mother had not yet seen the baby. She wondered if she could take the baby over to her parent's house on Mother's Day. I cautioned her about this, but felt that since she remained well for such a long period of time, it sounded reasonable to take a chance. This was before I was told during sleep that initial contact should be brief and must be preceded with education of patient and family, and that it was necessary to provide careful monitoring over the next several days.

We met shortly thereafter, and something occurred that was so startling and puzzling that I did not think to look for subtle signs. An infant is far more attuned than we are to subtle changes in the mother. As soon as this patient arrived, she set her one-and-a-half-year-old baby on the floor, and instantly it raced across the room to me and started speaking in tongues. This was in the early 1970s and I never had heard anyone speaking in tongues, but it sounded like the baby was speaking some kind of language and was jabbering away in a very excited and concerned fashion. I sensed that the baby was trying to convey an important message concerning her mother, but the speaking in tongues distracted me from checking the mother more carefully for subtle signs of a return to infant mind.

Her visit with her parents was a very pleasant and enjoyable one; but after another day or two, her condition suddenly worsened, and the next week, she described her husband to me once more for the same four months. This time she described him as being a cruel, hostile person who beat her up and tormented the child. This was the same man she had described in glowing terms for the same time interval, but now he was seen through the eyes of the infant. Obviously she had been hurt in some way as an infant and experienced her main caretaker as being cruel and sadistic. Whatever originally happened could have been totally innocent, but now when she was re-experiencing all of her environment through the eyes of the infant, she saw her husband—the most important person in the world to her—as being cruel and sadistic.

I immediately hospitalized this woman, and the nurses refused to give her medication, believing she was well; and they wondered why I didn't hospitalize her husband instead. It did not take long for them to recognize her illness because she rapidly deteriorated until the medication was forthcoming.

A Third Important Treatment Principle

If there is a third major treatment principle beyond correct understanding and total separation, it is to do whatever helps the person move from infant to adult mind and brain, and nothing that causes movement in the opposite direction.

Our aim in psychotherapy is to get the person out of the infant mind and brain as fast as possible, as completely as possible, and for as long as possible.

What Causes Movement from Adult to Infant?

1. Contact with original nuclear family prior to full recovery, lengthy stabilization, and education of patient and family.
2. Failure or rejection such as caused by entering a university when not yet ready and the likelihood of failure is great, or entering a relationship that is destined to fail.
3. Criticism. We can never improve on a person by tearing that person down. Even helpful suggestions can be taken by the infant mind to mean disapproval. Any suggestions must follow statements of approval and recognition for work well done. Even then, suggestions

are better put in the form of a question as to whether something would be helpful.
4. The therapist and mental health worker must not relate to the patient as parent to infant. Speaking baby talk to the patient is taboo. The patient should learn to recognize this type of verbal interaction and know how to tactfully not permit it. Crayons and coloring books are not part of adult interests and giving these to a patient conveys the wrong message. It infantilizes the patient. The relationship should be kept adult to adult. A nurse in a group home, for example, said to a patient, "I'm going to take you shopping tomorrow." We *take* children to the store. How much better it would have been to say, "Let's go shopping together tomorrow." These subtleties are overlooked because the patient partly is the infant, which makes it seem natural to relate this way—but it is counterproductive. It keeps the patient in infant mind and brain. The infant mind will try to draw you into that kind of relationship to make you into the parent, but this the therapist must avoid.

What Causes Movement from Infant to Adult?

1. Total separation from original nuclear family, at least until the patient is solidly back on track for a long-enough period of time to achieve independence, self-sufficiency, a circle of friends, and stable employment.
2. Support at a distance makes this movement possible. Financial needs must be met during the recovery process. An atmosphere must be created that is conducive for growth and movement toward independence. Separation does not mean having the person live on the street. The patient should have an apartment or a group home and a well-structured plan that includes becoming financially independent. Finances can be handled first by covering basic expenses and then supplying automatic bank drafts on a daily basis, progressing to a weekly basis as the person learns to manage funds. If the person runs out of food because of careless spending, starvation will not occur when funds are provided on a daily or every other day or weekly basis. Since this is structured in advance, the person will learn to budget gradually without feeling rejected if they run out of funds for a day or two.

3. A treatment environment that allows for growth and development—which encourages physical, mental, emotional and spiritual development; education, learning a trade or a profession, studying music and the arts, becoming knowledgeable about current events, developing hobbies and interests and recreational activities; and learning to socialize.
4. Work is a very important part of recovery. When the patient is able, work should begin. This demands a daily structure and routine of keeping on a schedule. This is one of the most critical elements for getting back on track. It is a responsible adult function. Even before the patient is capable of independent living and going to work, small work tasks can be assigned, on a schedule, to help orient and prepare the patient for a future job.
5. Individual and group psychotherapy, but with people who understand serious disorders and who treat instead of drug the patient.

Chapter 15

Psychotherapy with Psychotic Patients

As with most other psychoses, treatment of schizophrenia should begin with a focus on problems of the earliest age of origin. If the person is psychotic and depressed, for example, the focus should be on the psychosis and not the depression. Many begin with a cocktail of several powerful mind-altering drugs, including antipsychotics, antidepressants, and antiseizure medications.

Even a person with no history of any mental or emotional disturbance would not be able to think clearly and function with such a mixture. If anything, this approach—while it quiets the mind—prevents higher-level function. The Second Annual Report of the King County, Washington State, Department of Human Services, revealed that in a survey of 9,302 mental health patients, over the course of one full year, only 5 of the 9,302 patients managed to find employment.

If there is an acute psychosis with depression, I might—for a short period of time—prescribe only an antipsychotic medication, just to help calm the person and enable the person to sleep. Sleep is very important for restoration of the mind. It is much easier to reason with a patient who is stabilized and rested. But medication is not the answer for getting the person well.

One particularly effective approach I've used, even in the first few minutes with the patient, is to say, for example, "Something happened to you at age fourteen months" (or whatever the age of origin appears to be).

This immediately catches the patient's attention of course, and if there is a younger sibling, it most likely was born at the age identified. It doesn't take long for a therapist to recognize age-of-origin using the five parameters described in previous chapters. Often only one parameter is evident, but one landmark might be all it takes. You tested yourself with the examples given in chapter 11 and saw how easy this sometimes can be.

If you are not comfortable making such a prediction at first, you at least can say (if there is a psychosis), "Something happened to you in the first two years of life" because in forty years, I have not identified an age-of-origin later than twenty-four months for psychosis. And if the person has flattened or inappropriate affect, you can be reasonably certain the original trauma was prior to eighteen months. Other parameters are outlined in the earlier chapters.

Birth of a sibling is one of the most common causes of schizophrenia. The separation from mother, produced by the birth of a sibling in the first eighteen months of life, resulted in a fivefold incidence of schizophrenia. Instead of one in a hundred, it was five in a hundred who developed the disorder. Remember the study with sixty halfway house patients? Seventeen had one sibling less than nineteen months younger, whereas only three of the "supernormal" group had a sibling in that age range-of-origin. A similar ratio was found in the previous hundreds we evaluated, and *birth-of-a-sibling is only one of thousands of possible infant separation traumas.*

When you are able to identify the specific age of origin, this confirmation is very convincing to the patient. It helps when explaining symptoms in terms of age-of-origin specificity.

When it is not the birth of a sibling, chances are the mother was ill or divorced, the family moved or some other calamity occurred. Perhaps an older child was deathly ill or had died. The patient will at least know if parents divorced or if one was drug or alcohol dependent or if a sibling died. Such confirmation also allows for a more convincing explanation of origin of the problem.

If the parents divorced when the child was three, you can be sure the mother was not happy and getting along with the husband when the patient was one or two.

With the identification of the cause of the patient's schizophrenia, it is easier for the patient to recognize and identify age-of-origin specific realities/feelings/behavior; and if the predicted age of origin matches the age at birth of a sibling, this helps the therapist gain confidence in his or her ability to identify age-of-origin. While birth of a sibling is not nearly as traumatic as death of the mother—or the mother going off to war—it is far more common and might still be the single most frequent cause.

After only a few minutes in the first interview, I explain the origin and mechanism to patients in a way that makes sense; and unless they are totally psychotic, they usually understand.

Even if the patient is hospitalized and acutely psychotic, I still begin the same way because often a very psychotic patient is able to understand. I always acknowledge that I absolutely believe the patient is experiencing everything exactly as the patient is describing it. I never doubt the truthfulness of what the patient says he or she is experiencing. This is important. We must begin with what the patient experiences to be real. We don't have to say that it *is* real, but we can say, "I know you are telling the truth about what you are experiencing. I have no doubt about that whatsoever."

Later in the first session, I might discuss various realities and note, "If you are dreaming and there is a bear chasing you, that is real until you wake up." Or "if you are hypnotized and told you are a rooster, that is real until the hypnotist snaps his fingers." Similarly, if a person shifts to a reality of the first year of life and uses the same brain cells he or she was using at the time, that is real too but at an earlier time. It can be likened to dreaming with eyes open.

I continue with "If ten people witness the same event, they experience it ten different ways. If one person experiences the same event at ten different ages, that person experiences it ten different ways." Then I might get into a discussion of various realities other patients have had, stemming from traumas at specific months during infancy. Still this is not challenging what the patient experiences, it is just opening up more possibilities.

I often ask, "What would you have said ten years ago if a man told you aliens had implanted something in his brain and were monitoring and controlling everything he did?" I actually use whatever delusion the patient is experiencing, and usually the patient responds truthfully and acknowledges that ten years ago, he or she would have said the person is crazy. Then I can explain that the other person had shifted to the age when the infant experiences most intensely the reality that everything is monitored and controlled (age thirteen to fifteen months).

Engaging the patient in real activities also is particularly helpful. Many years ago, a high school friend appeared at my door in a very psychotic and delusional state. My immediate response was, "Joe, let's go fishing." It just happened that the mackerel were running off the New Jersey shore, and the school was 110 miles long and 10 miles wide. It wasn't long before we began pulling them in, three or four or five at a time. It was very exciting, and soon the delusions were gone. He was back in the real world, or more specifically, back in the here and now—the current adult reality.

Any activity that a highly delusional patient can do should be encouraged. Maybe it is only sweeping the floor, but that is reality orienting. I have had psychotic patients chauffeur me to meetings or even navigate a boat for me from Philadelphia to Atlantic City.

It also is true that the mind focuses on the point in time where there is the most imminent threat to survival. If the greatest threat to a person's survival is in the seventeen-month-old-infant mind, then the person is guided by the reality of the seventeen-month-old mind.

Reality can shift to the present when a threat in the present is greater than that from infancy. One recovered schizophrenic described his own means of coming out of delusional reality by mounting a fast horse, racing through the woods, and hanging on for dear life. This put the immediate danger in the here and now, not during infancy. In France, during WW II, the asylum doors were opened and the patients were told "The Germans are coming and they are going to kill you." Even the most insane began to function. This undoubtedly is a factor as to why shock treatment works. This puts the fear in the present reality of the adult mind and brain. It might also be one reason why the old dunking chairs worked.

With the hospitalized patient who is coming out of a delusional system, there is an extraordinary but fleeting opportunity to make interpretations. It is an opportunity that must not be missed. This even holds true when the patient is receiving shock treatment. It is common practice to wait until the course of treatment is over prior to beginning psychotherapy, reasoning that the patient will forget everything anyway. But this logic causes the therapist to miss an extraordinary opportunity for interpretation, and this must not happen.

Every psychoanalyst knows that an interpretation must be made at the level in which the reality is being experienced; otherwise it is ineffective. The same applies during the short interval when the psychotic is beginning to come out of psychosis. An interpretation might be, "Yesterday you experienced the reality that those people were following you, and today you do not experience this to be so. Do you suppose that tomorrow what you experience to be real will change still further? It is critical that the patient be aware of this changing reality. This also is when the patient can really begin to understand the origin of the earlier reality. An example of a useful interpretation might be, "When first learning to walk, the whole world, which to the infant is mother, follows you everywhere so you don't fall down the stairs or put hairpins in the electrical outlets, etc."

Eventually, the psychotic reality becomes like that of a person who has a nightmare ten nights in a row until one night during the dream, they realize, "Oh, I've been here before. This is just a dream." This process of identifying earlier reality is what must occur with the psychotic. He or she must become familiar with the delusions, so if they should start to recur, the patient immediately can see the therapist and possibly even start taking medication for a while.

Therapeutic Alliance

A critical aspect of treatment is the development of a strong therapeutic alliance. This can occur in part through befriending the patient and interacting with the patient in the patient's own environment. The patient must come to regard the therapist as a friend who wants to help and who is not critical. A high degree of trust must develop—a trust that the therapist will accept the patient and will understand the patient's sensitivities and act accordingly. Ultimately, the therapist becomes the patient's anchor in reality to the extent that upon just seeing the therapist—even while in a delusional state—the patient reconnects with the treatment sessions and the reality they already established.

In the case of the woman who recovered following separation from her mother and then stormed out of the synagogue screaming and hallucinating when her mother walked in and sat next to her, a strong therapeutic alliance had developed—partly through interacting with her in her own environment. We almost never met at the office. The doctor-patient relationship in the office sometimes is too similar to a parent-infant relationship, which we try to avoid with a psychotic patient. Instead we would go shopping together or feed the cats in her apartment, and often we would meet at a fast-food restaurant for lunch. There is more privacy in a restaurant than in a psychiatrist's office. No one suspects it is a psychiatric session with a doctor, and the atmosphere is a normal part of everyday life.

It is critical not to move into a parent-infant relationship with the patient. The patient has ways of making the therapist a replacement for the parent and unconsciously tries to draw the therapist into such a relationship. One time, for example, this patient ordered just a carton of milk, and she did not even open the container. This was an attempt of the infant part of her mind to get me to take the role of a parent and say, "Drink your milk." Instead I ignored the fact that she did not drink her milk. I did not even ask, "Are you trying to get me to say drink your milk?" Another time, she did the same by ordering coleslaw and not touching it. Once more, I did not step into the parent-to-infant role.

She participated in group therapy that we called "the trap group." Every patient understood the trap of schizophrenia and learned to recognize when someone made even a slight shift into infant mind/brain/reality/behavior. They became very attuned to this phenomenon. On Wednesdays, all of us went together to the New Jersey shore to go fishing on a private boat; and afterward, we would stop for supper before returning home.

It is important to get the patient involved with normal activities of everyday living, encourage adult function and not reinforce the infant mind. The activity can be any adult activity that is good clean fun. It also can be a work activity, such as weeding the garden or putting up a fence. Sometimes that's not a good idea. One catatonic patient stood motionless, holding a posthole digger in hand, in my front yard, for more than two hours.

It is important not to speak baby talk to the patient or to infantilize the patient in any way. The relationship must be kept in the adult-to-adult mode. One time when providing a consultation with a patient at a university medical center in Philadelphia, the patient understood perfectly well the origin and mechanism of his disorder in the first ten minutes. He listened intently, and it was clear that he understood everything. Then the professor spoke baby talk to him. Instantly he shifted to the infant mind and understood nothing.

The larger part of the psychiatric community does not recognize relating parent to infant, and this only serves to perpetuate the disorder.

Chapter 16

Other Treatment Modalities

There are many factors that enhance recovery, and we should make use of any that we can. Here we present more than a dozen other treatment modalities. Some apply more to persons with depression than with schizophrenia, but persons with schizophrenia become depressed too. All examples add to your overall knowledge and understanding.

<u>Love Energy</u>

The enhancement of love energy applies to everyone, even to those without a diagnosable disorder. Learning to increase love while diminishing need and nonforgiveness is perhaps the most important factor in all healing: physical, mental, emotional, and spiritual.

With a depressed person, for example, what happens when the person falls in love? Immediately the depression is gone! What about the so-called chemical imbalance and the serotonin deficiency? Are these but mythical creations? Certainly, the depressed person who falls in love was not suddenly given more serotonin or a reuptake inhibitor. Yet the change is dramatic.

One can cure depression with this approach alone. You simply cannot be in love and depressed at the same time. The opposite of love is need or desire, and sometimes the two are confused because both are very intense feelings, but they are not difficult to distinguish because the by-product of love is happiness, and the by-product of need is unhappiness. Therefore, you can know by the fruit. It is *selfless* love that is incongruous with depression. And there are many ways to develop and enhance this love energy, other than through romance and all of its hurdles, traps, and pitfalls. This is a major dimension of treatment for any depression. And it helps very much in the treatment of schizophrenia too because movement from need to love is movement from the infant to the adult, which is the direction necessary for permanent recovery.

Love energy is such an important dimension of treatment that we devote an entire chapter to it.

The opposite of love is need or desire. When needs are not met, the needs can turn to anger. A therapist can bring a person out of depression by demanding more and more. This stirs anger instead of love, but at least there is movement. Depression is anger turned toward the self, and the patient cannot be angry and depressed at the same time. Make sure it is not a family member stirring the anger. That will only send the EE factor off the scale and make the depression worse. It must be a therapist.

I prefer enhancing love. There are other occasions when love can be precipitated by triggering need. This works in a need-oriented or even an apathetic relationship. In Christianity, particular note is paid to the fact that Christ said he preferred people hot or cold, but not lukewarm. Hot would be equivalent to love, cold equivalent to need, and lukewarm equivalent to apathy. The route from apathy to love sometimes is through need. A secret formula is to trigger need *but prevent all hurt and jealous feelings*. This can result in intense love when a relationship has become distant and apathetic. This is explained in chapter 18 on love energy.

Another treatment modality for depression is light therapy. This is the administration light, in measured units called lux. This has been well advertised because of its commercial interests, and by now most have heard of this. It definitely has value. In the fall and winter months, when it is darker in the northern hemisphere, persons are more likely to become depressed, and depressed people seem to like darkness. In fact, they prefer darkened rooms; but when exposed to bright lights, they are less depressed. In recent decades, measurements have been made to determine the optimal amount required for beneficial purposes. But this is only one of many factors; and I simply recommend that depressed individuals replace lightbulbs with 150 watt bulbs or, if they can afford it, take a vacation to the tropics. Everyone feels better in a nice tropical resort where the sun shines all day.

There is nothing wrong with getting a lux lamp and sitting in front of ten thousand lux for half an hour every day, but this is not to be used to the exclusion of the many other treatment modalities.

Those who experience springtime mania have to reverse this procedure and wear dark sunglasses in the springtime. A related condition, opposite end of the spectrum, opposite remedy.

So far, the dimensions we have touched upon are (1) correct understanding, which is critical for a more permanent recovery from any disorder. (2) Separation from people, places, and things that draw us into the past—into early infant mind and brain. This means a total separation from original nuclear family members with not even a brief telephone call until independent and solidly stabilized for a long-enough period of time. This alone can end an intractable depression or psychosis. Sometimes the acute illness will disappear within days or weeks. Then we touched upon (3) the enhancement of love because you cannot be in love and feel depressed at the same time. This is a major treatment modality to which an entire chapter is devoted.

The fourth modality we discussed is light treatment, which can be beneficial, especially in those cases of depression or mania that are more seasonal. A fifth factor or treatment modality is macrobiotic diet, which gives more energy and therefore a greater sense of well-being. One criterion for depression is loss of energy. A healthy diet produces enormous levels of energy and also provides mental clarity.

A sixth treatment factor would be proper exercise—and especially aerobic exercise, which improves health, causing persons to feel more invigorated, more energetic, and therefore feeling better. This helps, and it can be an important factor for countering depression. Stretching exercises lead to greater flow of energy and clarity of mind, and brain exercise is particularly helpful in schizophrenia as persons return to the adult mind and brain, which have been relatively less active during the course of the illness. The patient must not only return to the adult brain structures, but he or she must begin exercising those structures as well—very much in the same way a person who has spent a year in a coma would have to exercise the legs before regaining the ability to walk. As the person reaches a sufficient degree of recovery and stabilization, it is good to encourage the patient to take college courses, gradually at first, in a way that does not risk failure or rejection. Learning must be interactive, not merely watching educational TV. A chimpanzee can do that.

A seventh factor is sleep. Too often, this is overlooked. At times, proper rest alone can bring a person out of psychosis. The mind is clearer, and persons feel better. As simple as this sounds, it is true. Physically, persons are healthier and are better able to function. They can do more and they feel better about themselves. Some bipolar patients can be kept from manic episodes by simply using an appropriate amount of medication to achieve adequate sleep.

The eighth approach is through meditation and learning to think and to function at a slower brain wave frequency. This is another major approach that we hear very little about in psychotherapy. For this reason, we include a small chapter on meditation.

With meditation, a person is more relaxed. When there is less stress and worry, there is less attention focused on the self and "what's going to happen to me?" Therefore there is less depression because there is less energy focused back to the self. Learning to think and to use the mind at meditative levels is beneficial for countless purposes in addition to relaxation: it is utilized for decision making, finding answers to problems, habit control, and also as a reality check. Delusional systems sometimes do not exist in a meditative state. Patients can control how they feel throughout each day by spending a few minutes in meditation and picturing themselves remaining more relaxed and at peace throughout the entire day. This is something like self-hypnosis. It takes only a few minutes to do, and it is very easy to learn. A most effective level for this purpose is just slightly more relaxed than our usual wide-awake state. It is the level of relaxation found in nature—for example, if one were to sit quietly, alone, in a deep forest. Anyone can learn to reach this state in a brief period of time. You can learn how in the next chapter—and then apply it any time, at will, for your own personal use.

A ninth treatment modality is work, particularly in the area of helping others. Depressed people must help others. Loving, caring, doing, and helping others is the correct direction of flow of love energy; and it is incongruous with depression. This is a major treatment modality. Helping others enhances love energy. It can add enormously to one's sense of self-worth and feelings of well-being. Work is also reality orienting, and it helps bring persons out of psychosis.

A tenth dimension is through adding more meaning to life. This was pioneered by the late Dr. Viktor Frankl of Vienna. He called this logotherapy or existential analysis. In explaining his approach, Dr. Frankl's favorite example that he told over and over again was of a forced march during WW II from one SS camp to another, in which he didn't know if he, physically, would be able to cover the distance under the circumstances that prevailed—until he pictured himself lecturing to a group of students and telling them of his horrendous ordeal. He said that from that point forward, his journey became effortless. This is how logotherapy was born—a valuable approach, particularly with older adults whose children have left, whose friends have died, who no longer work, and for whom life no longer seems to have meaning.

Still his method was birthed out of ego need instead of love—but remember, hot or cold is better than lukewarm. Nothing is derived out of apathy. Love versus need is energy flowing outward vs. back to the self. Frankl's approach entails adding meaning to life, whether it is through love or through ego need. Need is far superior to apathy because once the energy is flowing, it can be turned quickly into love. While it is preferable to start with the intensification of love, it can begin with work that fills ego needs; and once the energy is flowing, it can turn to compassion and caring for the ones being helped, which is love.

Sometimes adding meaning can be very simple. Early in my career, I was called upon to see a man in a nursing home, who was so depressed he would not eat or get out of bed. When I asked him to get up, the nurse started to help him sit up. I said, "No, let him do it." Then the nurse started to button his shirt, and I said, "No, let him do that." It took a while, but he was able to do this small task which added a degree of dignity. Then I gave him the job of emptying the ashtrays and filling the water glasses at the nursing home. With just that much meaning added to his life, his depression disappeared within a few days. He was of importance to someone again.

A modern-day psychiatrist, treating strictly according to current protocol, would think first of the therapeutic indications and side-effect profile of various antidepressant medications. The next consideration would be the special needs of the elderly and would begin with the current philosophy of start low and go slow, which is correct when medicating a geriatric patient. If the first medication didn't work after one month, they would increase the dose; and if that didn't work, they would switch to another medication; and if that didn't work, they might again increase the dose, and the next step might be to add another drug. But this patient was well, practically overnight, and much quicker than medication ever could have worked. Not even shock treatment could have brightened him that fast. The irony of this miraculous recovery is that he was my very first patient in 1963 during my first year of psychiatry residency training at the Menninger School of Psychiatry. How far have we come and which direction did we go?

Notice anything different about the approach so far? Of the many dimensions for treatment mentioned so far, the only one we hear much about is the light therapy, and this perhaps is because it has become commercial. But there are many factors to consider, and for a disorder as serious as major depression or schizophrenia, we must take into account everything that contributes to the disorder and everything that can lead to a more full and permanent recovery.

Here is another novel approach that I have not seen in the literature or heard in the profession, but which is highly effective. We will call it treatment modality number 11. You have heard that anxiety is contagious. When you are with a person who is very anxious and restless, this has a carryover effect and causes you to be a little bit that way yourself. Depression is the same way. When you are depressed, other persons around you can feel a little blue. When I am with someone who is in a manic state, I find myself writing twice as fast. So feelings really *are* contagious. In a football stadium, you know what happens when the home team wins. The crowd goes wild. Likewise, if you are with a person who is in a state of absolute peace and bliss, these attributes have a powerful carryover effect too. The problem is you don't meet such people very often. So what I tried with a number of my patients was to have them listen to recordings of holy people who are in a state of absolute peace and bliss. Depressed patients who listened while in a relaxed state with eyes closed were not able to remain depressed. It didn't matter if they couldn't understand the words. The peace and bliss were transferred onto them. The transferring of peace and bliss was amazing and something that deserves careful research.

Meanwhile, this is something you can try. Any anointed spiritual music can do the same. It is best to listen with eyes closed. This eliminates 75 percent of external stimuli and reduces internal stimuli as well, so instead of listening with 10 percent of your attention, it is more like 90 percent. You will know the transfer of this peace and love by how you feel when you listen in a relaxed state with eyes closed. You will know by the fruit.

Now, of course, there are other treatment modalities; and we should consider all of them. For a severe suicidal depression that will not budge, shock treatment still is used. As a matter of fact, this is one of the quickest means of recovery from severe depression, and usually it has fewer side effects than long-term use of medication. Let's call this treatment modality number 12. I do not use this anymore, and have not used it for nearly twenty years, partly because my practice has changed; but on occasion when a person is so depressed that everything seems hopeless or when a person is in an intractable psychosis, this is something to consider. If persons are having bad dreams, you might shake them to awaken them. If they are delirious, you might slap their face to help bring them out of it. Similarly, if the person is caught in the depths of depression or psychosis, shock can bring them out of it quickly; and it certainly is less harmful than a lifelong course of powerful, mind-altering drugs. But *I would not use this if the person were to return to the same setting in which the major depressive or psychotic episode occurred.* Why use a drastic measure to get a person well and then return the person to the same environment in which the acute psychotic or major depressive episode occurred? This probably is why long-term outcome studies for shock treatment are poor.

All factors that move the person deeper into illness should be eliminated before launching drastic measures to bring the person back from the infant or toddler mind/brain/reality/feelings and behavior. Our treatment concept is to get the person out of the earlier mind/brain/reality as fast as possible, as completely as possible, and for as long as possible. A return to the surroundings and conditions that were in place prior to treatment would not be consistent with keeping the person well for as long as possible, and without first achieving a *sustained* recovery, the person remains too vulnerable to relapse.

For persons with depression related to grief over the loss of a loved one, another novel approach is the programmed dream, which we shall call treatment modality number 13. This is such an important dimension of treatment that we devote an entire chapter to it (chapter 19). This technique can end years of agony in a single night. *The person simply decides to have a dream about the lost loved one, decides that the dream will not be upsetting, and decides that the dream itself will resolve all upset feelings. The person then decides to awaken at the very end of the dream, remember it, and write it down.*

One patient, for example, grieved so much over the death of her mother that when I first saw her nine years after the loss, she still burst into tears every time she mentioned her mother. So I told her to have the dream as I just described. The very next week, when she told the dream, which was just a happy shopping trip with her mother, all the upset feelings were gone. No tears, no agony, none whatsoever. The very next week, her psychosomatic conditions began disappearing because they had related to guilt and unconscious self-punishment over the mother's death. It still is a mystery as to how her dream cured her long-standing grief reaction, but it did. Probably it instilled in her an absolute knowing that her mother is all right. Dreams often are more like visits, following which the dreamer *knows* that the lost loved one is OK.

Even a three-year-old was able to cure herself of a serious problem in a single night using the dream technique. She was taken from a cocaine-addicted mother at age two and placed in a foster home, but she was so frightened that she hid under their kitchen table and would not come out. Eventually she warmed up to her very loving foster parents, and then she became particularly fond of her foster daddy. He was the whole world to her. But when she was three, he died of lung cancer, and she was devastated. So I said to her, "You can visit your daddy any night you want during sleep. Tonight he is going to visit you and take away all your upset feelings." The very next morning, this little girl awakened, shouting, "Mommy, Mommy! Daddy brought me a baby doll last night." And before her mother could dissuade her, she popped out of bed, ran to the back corner of a closet, and dug out a little baby doll. She was a visitor in that house and might never have explored that closet. Some might even wonder if this was a visit from the spirit world. From then on, she carried that little doll everywhere she went, and the upset feelings were gone. That "dream" did more for her than years of child psychoanalysis, and any child analyst would understand why.

We get miracles, one after another, with programmed dreams. You can find solutions to the most difficult problems: medical, marital, financial, child rearing—any problem in life. There is no limit when we use this approach. It is a major treatment modality, so much so that we devote an entire chapter to it. It took many years to realize this provides the same miracle as what many describe as the miracle of prayer, but any night at will. In thirty-nine years, I have not known a person to receive a wrong answer, which indicates it must be coming from the highest source.

Anything following the programmed dream technique has to be anticlimactic, but there are still other modalities. The power therapies offer remarkable ways of removing resistance, removing blocks that prevent the release of conflicts of the past. We have seen the development of delayed posttraumatic stress disorders and how the defensive wall builds and thickens, year after year, in a lifelong process of protecting ego from overwhelming exposure to the repressed trauma and conflicts of the distant past. The power therapies provide a means of immediately disengaging the defensive wall and neutralizing the underlying trauma in the therapeutic setting. Sometimes huge conflicts are removed in minutes. Such modalities include thoughtfield therapy (TFT), emotional freedom technique (EFT), traumatic incident reduction (TIR), and eye movement trauma desensitization (EMD/R). One of the more promising of these is the recent emotional transformation therapy (ETT), which can quickly transform emotional states, bring forth insights and creativity, and even improve brain functioning. This can be an asset to psychotherapy and also help with medical problems.

There are various other enhancers for achieving deeper levels of relaxation such as with sound currents and frequencies, monochromatic light, magnetic therapy, brain gym, and other approaches for equalizing both halves of the brain. These assist in reaching deeper levels of consciousness, deeper states of relaxation, and better utilization of brain. The Life Program is one such modality that enables persons to reach slower brain wave frequencies within minutes, providing an effective means of relaxation and clarity of mind. These modalities, along with the power therapies, we will call treatment modality number 14.

For treatment modality number 15, let's consider medication. I know about medicines, I have studied many psychiatric medications including the major MAO inhibitors, the well-known tricyclics, the serotonin reuptake inhibitors, the atypicals, and the augmentors as well as the herbal remedies. Presently, I rarely use any of the antidepressants. For the psychoses, I am familiar with the antipsychotic medications too. I am not against a limited use of these medications. They can be helpful at times, but often their effectiveness is greatly overstated. Regrettably, not even a small fraction of what one pharmaceutical company pays for outcome studies on one medication is devoted to scientific testing of the usefulness of any of the methods described above.

I have no doubt about which is more effective. I have seen the results. If one treats the whole person and all aspects of the depression or schizophrenia instead of just medicating symptoms, it is very effective. Results often occur in a shorter period of time than required for medication to even begin to take effect.

After outlining the above fifteen modalities, working late into the night, I went to bed and began having a very ethereal dream. I didn't remember all of the dream, and I was having difficulty trying to analyze it; but while still asleep, I was simply told the interpretation: "With the first fourteen modalities, you didn't do a thing, you watered the garden," implying, "who made it grow?" The music, the meditation, the dreams, the love—these are modalities of the Spirit, and we just let the Spirit do the work. Picturing things better, picturing feeling better, knowing this is so is just allowing the Spirit to do the work.

Words spoken like this during sleep come at a speed of thought, and there never is an extra word. While the dream was not totally clear, the words remained indelibly etched in my mind and brain.

The next statement regarding the fifteenth treatment modality really startled me. It came in words I am not accustomed to saying. What I was told was, "Medications are of Satan, derived strictly out of greed, out of desire for power, desire for money: lies in the research; lies in the marketing; targeting the weak, the infirm, the unsuspecting, and the disabled." Those words were spoken with great power and authority.

Wow! I never would be so bold and accusatory. That hit me like a bombshell. I am not that way with words, but Truth is unbending.

In considering the facts, there are hard-data, evidence-based research outcome studies confirming what I was told. We already mentioned the King County, Department of Community and Human Services, Ordinance No. 13974, Second Annual Report. This revealed that out of 9,302 mental health patients, over the course of one full year, only 5 recovered well enough to find a menial job. The cost for that year was over 90 million dollars, and we know what comprised the main treatment. It was medication, extolled as being the only thing proven, in double-blind, placebo-controlled, hard-data, evidence-based outcome studies—conducted by pharmaceutical companies and approved by the Food and Drug Administration. (Note: I must commend King County for their scientific integrity in publishing the second annual report. Even though scientists are obligated to publish all studies that are not pilot studies, pharmaceutical companies often maintain secrecy regarding unfavorable outcomes.)

Third world countries, without modern medications, have a greater rate of recovery from serious mental and emotional disorders, and in a 1967 NIMH research study of 299 hospitalized mental patients, half were given placebo and the other half given one of three antipsychotic medications. The researchers were trying to determine which neuroleptic drug was most effective. The results shocked them. What they discovered was that in each instance, the placebo had a better outcome. This was reported in the *American Journal of Psychiatry*, Vol. 123 (1967), 986-995. Even though the findings were conclusive, the researchers would not recommend giving a placebo! Why?

Since the 1967 study, we have heard repeatedly that the newer medications are more effective and have fewer side effects. This has been the steady mantra for the last forty years. But then an independent study, testing the newer antipsychotic medications against the older ones, revealed they were not any better. The only things bigger and better were the costs and the claims. Indeed, they targeted the weak and the infirm, told them lies, and gouged them unmercifully.

These studies and many others support my clinical assessment of psychotropic medications over the course of many years, and they confirm what I was told during sleep.

When I turned on the television later that same day, following what I was told during sleep, the very first words I heard were: "Book of Revelation 18:23: 'And the light of a candle shall shine no more at all in you . . . for by your sorceries were all nations deceived.'" The Greek word that was translated as "Sorcery" is translated from the Greek word *pharmakeia*—which refers to the preparation or the use of drugs!

I took this as confirmation of what I was told during sleep. What incredible synchronicity! What is the probability of turning on the TV the same day and at the precise moment and the particular channel where that person was uttering those exact words and following the words that were told to me during sleep? It could be coincidence. Everything could be coincidence. But for all such experiences to be coincidental seems less probable than not. There comes a point where even the skeptic must begin to be skeptical about his or her own skepticism. For some, that endpoint is infinity.

This does not mean that anyone should suddenly stop taking medication. That could be dangerous. Each individual must consult with his or her own physician before attempting to change any medication that has been prescribed. This is a decision to be made between patient and treating physician. Most physicians know that reducing medication must be done gradually, over a period of time, usually no more than 3 to 10 percent per week. The SSRIs are particularly dangerous to taper because persons stop producing their own serotonin and can become suicidal. Ten grams daily of fish oil should be supplemented immediately with psychotic and depressed patients. That's only a tablespoonful, and it is not a chemical; it is completely natural. Harvard University used fourteen grams. This at least reduces the need for medication or eliminates the need altogether. It helps overcome psychosis, anxiety, depression, and bipolar disorder. It might be the most effective oral remedy there is for bipolar disorder. The primary side effect is that it lowers cholesterol level and reduces the chance of a heart attack.

Chapter 17

Meditation

One of the most effective states of consciousness for problem solving and decision making is a light level of meditation—often referred to as an alpha brain wave frequency. Although deep levels of meditation are beneficial for other purposes, it doesn't require more than a light level of meditation to achieve effective treatment of certain mental and emotional disorders.

Ordinarily, patients can learn techniques of light meditation in a relatively short period of time. When going to a meditation level with the therapist, it is not uncommon for a patient to arrive at answers and reach decisions very quickly. Many of the following light meditation techniques are taught quite effectively in the Silva Method course.

The light level of meditation is, perhaps, the optimum level of consciousness that people have used for thousands of years. It is only slightly more relaxed than our usual wide-awake state. It is the level we reach while in the peace and tranquility found in nature, which we might attain while just sitting in a deep woods and listening—with eyes closed—to the sounds and the stillness of the forest. It is not the usual level we experience in urban life, with the distractions of bright lights, loud noises, and pressures of modern society.

There are various ways to reach this state. One method is to sit comfortably, preferably not leaning over, because that requires muscle tension. Just sit well balanced. The spine will straighten and elongate as you move into meditation and experience an enhanced flow of energy.

Unless you were reared in a country without chairs or have practiced yoga for many years, the effort to meditate in the lotus position might be counterproductive. By the time we raise our legs to the level we are sitting, the lower back tilts and produces stress and discomfort, which is not conducive for meditation. The idea is to sit comfortably, totally balanced, in a posture that is not difficult to maintain. This reduces discomfort that could distract you.

The patient needs to be assured this is not hypnosis. It is the patient directing his or her own mind to do what he or she wishes to do for beneficial purposes. It is merely getting to a more relaxed state of mind. A level that is superior for clarity of mind, memory, and decision making—a level more open to the spirit. The therapist simply acts as a guide in this process, and the therapist can go to the same level of consciousness with the patient.

It is helpful to elevate the gaze approximately fifteen or twenty degrees. When people try to recall or think about something, their eyes automatically turn upward. This alone helps a person reach an alpha brain wave frequency. So we make use of this in our light meditation. Allow the gaze to move upward and then gradually allow the eyelids to drop. This level of meditation is reached with eyes closed.

From there the process of going to a light level of meditation is fairly simple. We take in a deep breath and count exhalations, from ten to zero, telling ourselves we are going to a deeper level of consciousness, deeper all the time, deeper and deeper, approaching the most effective level of mind, more relaxed all the time, and any such similar words you choose. Decide in advance that any extraneous sounds, such as the telephone ringing, will only cause you to go deeper.

If we begin to think about a problem when we reach this light level of meditation, we are no longer there. *Therefore we formulate the question in advance* and tell ourselves that the very moment we reach zero, the first thought will be the answer to whatever question we have formulated. Sometimes the answer will pop in prior to reaching zero. That is OK. You will learn to recognize how the answer arrives and learn to trust in the answer you receive, more all the time, as you repeatedly receive enlightened answers.

It matters not what the question is, as long as it is not counter to the laws of morality and justice, or is not a foolish question—such as "what is going to happen?"—because regardless what is going to happen, you still need to know what to do. The patient is encouraged to formulate a question for which he needs an answer. Perhaps it is a question about a child or a spouse or perhaps a question about a job or a school or about a financial or a medical problem. Or it can be a simple matter such as what to buy at the supermarket or selecting the right outfit to wear to a party. Pick anything and decide that when you reach zero, the first thing that occurs will be the best answer. When I do this with a patient, and we both program to receive the answer to the patient's question, almost always we reach the same answer—even though neither one of us might have considered the particular answer in advance.

When the patient has received the answer while still at a light level of meditation, this is an opportunity to reinforce how much better the patient feels. The sense of well-being is usually superior to the effects of any medication. It takes only minutes to achieve and the patient feels much better. Once the person has received the answer to the question formulated in advance, there is still more benefit to be derived from being in a light meditation. The person can picture remaining in the relaxed state throughout the entire day and can visualize going through all the daily activities at this level of peace and tranquility. If the person is worried about a job interview or a performance, the person can conjure up a mental image of the actual event while in the relaxed state and see everything going well, *with the interviewer or the audience being well pleased.* This will improve outcome because anxiety is less and the performance superior when the patient already mentally has done the task well in the relaxed state. The results can be so dramatic that we wonder if we influenced the minds of the audience in advance. Those who believe in prayer are more likely to consider this possibility and might choose to combine the meditation with prayer.

So we begin by preparing the patient as described above and asking the patient to formulate a question for which an answer will occur when they reach zero or anywhere along the way. Have the patient decide that any extraneous sounds will only cause him or her to go deeper.

Then have the patient sit comfortably, elevate the gaze slightly, allow the eyelids to close, and begin counting exhalations, slowly, from ten to zero, telling the self they are going deeper and deeper, approaching the most effective level of mind.

By using more parameters, we can make the technique even more effective. So not only do we count backward from ten to zero, telling ourselves that we are going deeper all the time, but we coordinate this with breathing. We inhale slowly, and as we exhale, we mentally see and hear the number 10. If it is difficult to picture the number, then just imagine the number. That's OK.

You also can picture going down a flight of stairs, as you count backward from ten to zero, telling yourself that you are going deeper all the time, approaching your most effective level of consciousness. Don't question this. When you get to zero, you will be at a deeper level of consciousness. Guaranteed. You already are at a deeper level when you just close your eyes.

Decide that your mind will reach its most effective level, and presume it will do so. It knows how. That is the level where for thousands of years we have functioned best. Does a fish need to learn how to swim or a rabbit how to hop? Trust your mind will do this and it will. The human mind has done this for thousands of years.

When you reach zero and receive the answer, this is the time to note how much better you feel, and it is the time to direct your mind to do what you want it to do. In this way you achieve a dual purpose with your meditation.

You can also repeat the process to get further clarification and elaboration regarding the answer you received. If patient and therapist are doing this together, this second time through, each might count from ten to zero silently; and then after receiving the answer, neither one speaks until the other's eyes are open. You would not want to interrupt the process when the other person is still counting and going deeper.

Clinical Examples

A twenty-one-year-old man had an extreme conflict that caused him to be suicidal. He was caught in great conflict with his father. The father promised he never would do what his father had done to him. He was going to leave his fortune to this young man, unlike his own father who had left him with nothing.

Unfortunately, this lad's father had only his own father for a teacher. He had promised a large inheritance plus a pension that just went on from generation to generation. Promises were made throughout this young man's early life; promises that would not be kept. As his father's life was coming to an end, it was revealed that his father had sold his pension fund for a meager amount, cashed in his life insurance policies, and even gambled away all of this young man's college funds!

So this young man was torn by strong feelings of murderous rage toward his father, coupled with equal feelings of love because his father had been his idol. He was experiencing deception of the highest magnitude from the person he trusted the most.

Consequently he was extremely depressed; he was punching holes in walls and driving his car 100 mph. He did not know whether to kill the father or commit suicide, and he was at a point where he might do either.

After he vented and described this situation in great detail, I suggested the simple relaxation technique and told him that as soon as we reached zero, the first thing that would occur would be exactly what to do.

Minutes later, he had the clear awareness that he must cut all ties with his father, forget him, and eliminate him from his life altogether. There was no doubt in this. Apart from his father, this was a healthy twenty-one-year-old man who was getting all As in college, who would be able to work and earn enough to start school in the fall and who would be a total success in life.

His problem was resolved that fast. He looked deeply relaxed compared to the extreme stress associated with the life-and-death matters he had presented minutes earlier.

This is the light meditation level I used when I received the incredible vision of the Trinity ring after being directed by the Spirit to meditate. It also is what I used when I was directed to meditate on what is God and found the answer waiting for me one minute later (love, energy, the creative force.) So this technique can be used to receive answers directly from a higher Source. Christians identify this source as the Holy Spirit. Regardless how you conceptualize this source, once you begin to use this means of attaining information and guidance on a regular basis and begin receiving its guidance, you likely will begin to recognize that this source of knowledge is beyond the technology and limits of man. We can access this source even with just the light level of meditation described in this chapter.

This meditation technique is effective for finding answers and for helping patients beyond difficult situations. It is a wonderful technique for patients who procrastinate and have difficulty making decisions. Tell them: "When you reach zero, your first thought will be the answer." This works! And they *will* have a first thought.

Lastly, this level of consciousness can be used for habit control. One time I wanted to stop eating candy, so I pictured a bowl of candy at this level and placed a big black X across the image. There was no more desire for candy. Six months later, when coming out of a restaurant, I started to put my hand in the bowl of mints. Immediately I saw the image with the black X across it, and all desire was gone. This light level of meditation is extremely effective.

For a deeper level of relaxation, here is another simple exercise. It is one that I enjoy doing with patients because the peace and tranquility lingers throughout the remainder of the day.

The most difficult thing to do with this exercise is to maintain awareness and not fall asleep. In meditation, we aim for deeper relaxation but heightened awareness. This translates into slower brain wave frequencies but with greater amplitude. Usually when we relax, we are falling asleep. So now we must train ourselves to go to two seemingly opposite directions at once.

In this particular meditation exercise we move our awareness to different parts of the body. First, we place our awareness at the top of the head, a little spot at the very crown of the head. Then we move our awareness to the center of the forehead until we become aware of a warmth and a tingling sensation there.

It does not matter which sequence you use, but for this example, we will move from there to bridge of nose, to left eye, to bridge of nose, to right eye, to bridge of nose, to tip of nose, to left cheek, to left ear, to left cheek, to tip of nose, to right cheek, to right ear, to right cheek, to tip of nose, to lips, to tip of the tongue, to root of tongue, to tip of tongue, to lips, to chin, to throat, to center of chest (heart), to left shoulder, to left elbow, to left wrist, to left little finger, to ring finger, to middle finger, to index finger, to thumb, to wrist, to elbow, to shoulder, to center of chest, to right shoulder, to right elbow, to right wrist, to little finger, to ring finger, to middle finger, to index finger, to thumb, to wrist, to elbow, to shoulder, to center of chest, to upper abdomen, to umbilicus, to lower abdomen, to left hip, to thigh, to knee, to ankle, to left small toe, to the next toe, to the next, to the next, and to the big toe. Then back to the ankle, to the knee, to the hip and back to the center of the lower abdomen, to the right hip, to the right knee, to ankle, to right small toe, to the next toe, to the next, to the next, and to the big toe. Then back to the ankle, to the knee, to the hip and back to the center of the lower abdomen, to the umbilicus, to the upper abdomen, to the center of the chest, to the throat, to the chin, to the lips, to the nose, to the center of the forehead, to the top of the head. Then we feel the awareness moving downward—like a water level—one millimeter at a time and out the fingertips and the toes.

This can be embellished along the way by such things as exploring the eye socket, noticing the coolness of the breath across the nostrils, the moisture/dryness in the lips, the position of the tongue, the enhanced auditory acuity when focusing on the root of the tongue, becoming aware of the heart beating in the center of the chest, the position of the fingers, etc. It is important to place awareness with each area of focus, feeling warmth or a tingling sensation. One can ad lib or embellish the flow of this awareness freely.

The challenge is to stay awake during this exercise. When you practice this, you might find that you remain more at peace and tranquil throughout the remainder of the day.

The person who showed me this was Swami Rama. Elmer Green, the grandfather of biofeedback, tested Swami Rama and noted he was not able to do everything he claimed—when subjected to the confines of an experimental laboratory—but he could do many things that were quite remarkable.

The first technique I described, for a light level of meditation, is similar to what I learned from Mr. Jose Silva, in the Silva Mind training program. He was a very unique man who never spent one day in school—but he taught 25 million people how to use the mind! One night he became so frustrated while studying psychology books, that he threw them on the ground and decided to abandon his pursuit. That very night, according to Silva, he had an apparition or vision of Christ, and was given a clear sign that caused him to forge ahead. I became his psychiatric consultant from 1971 until his passing in 1999.

Although I do not use or endorse all that was taught in that training program, there are parts of it that can be quite effective, and I found it to be very worthwhile. The course proposed to teach psychic diagnosis, guaranteeing full refund if the person was not convinced of clairvoyance by the end of the week. All had opportunity to test themselves at the end of the course by trying psychic diagnoses. Each was given name, age, location of several persons with medical problems while at the relaxed level of consciousness, and then asked to identify the medical problem. The results were such that no one asked for a refund.

Jose Silva said that the approach was effective because it was used for the purpose of helping the other person: it was used to diagnose and then to treat through visualizing the person well and the illness leaving. This explanation is in keeping with the correct direction of flow of love energy. Dr. Carl Simonton developed from this a means of cancer treatment through visualization and reported many successful cases.

Perhaps all such training programs are stepping stones for further development. This was my first introduction to spiritual life in 1969.

Deep Meditation/God-consciousness

We cannot even begin to delve into practices of deep meditation here, but we can mention a few general concepts. We must not overlook deep meditation. There are many benefits to be derived. You might think you don't have time to learn deep meditation. Truth is, time becomes available. All that is required is your commitment—real commitment—to your own well-being, and time will become your servant rather than your master. To some extent, it can replace sleep because you learn to achieve a state of deep relaxation. A good time to meditate might be when you awaken in the middle of the night. You are already at a very deep level and the body still is asleep. Try meditating at this level before you even move. Become alert while remaining totally relaxed.

For deep meditation, we think of mind/body/spirit, mind/body/soul, or mind/body/God. All meditation practices begin with mind. This includes the position in which one sits, the breathing techniques, and the special body postures that enhance our ability to meditate. The first aim of meditation is to quiet the mind, to limit our busy thinking machines—where ten thoughts are connected to ten more to ten more, etc.—causing the mental chatter to continue unceasingly.

Since we can think only one thought at a time, we can still the mind by bringing it to a single point of focus by staring at a candle flame or focusing on breathing or on a sound current, a pattern or any single thing or concept. If you are spiritual, you can repeat whatever name you use for God. Stilling the mind takes much practice because the mind is not easy to subdue. Any of these approaches will bring the mind to a single point of focus.

Once the mind is quieted and the individual is able to focus on a single point, it is then possible to shut off that single point of attention and transcend "body/mind/brain/thought" and move closer to God-consciousness. Holding the breath for just a short while can enhance this transition.

We must not minimize what people are able to do through the utilization of deep meditation practices, when combined with saintly virtues and aspirations. Continuous expressions of devotional love, praise, and worship throughout all waking moments, when combined with obedience to higher direction given, is key to greater development. This enhances the ability to love and to reach states of enlightenment that surpass worldly knowledge.

Chapter 18

Love Energy: The Life Force and The Fountain of Youth

Proper nutrition, exercise, and relaxation are recognized as vital ingredients for a long and healthy life. But a fourth ingredient, LOVE, can add as much to one's energy and longevity as all other factors combined; and yet this important factor is all but omitted from current health protocols and even from scientific study.

While love's great power might be overlooked in modern science, it is not lost in scripture. For example, in Song of Solomon 8:6-7, "Set me as a seal upon thine heart, as a seal upon thine arm: for love is strong as death; its jealousy unyielding as the grave. It burns like blazing fire, like a mighty flame. Many waters cannot quench love; rivers cannot wash it away."

Love's powerful effects are noticed but not deciphered. Take for example a man who eats nothing but junk food, smokes, doesn't exercise, drinks beer, sports a potbelly, and leads a stressful life. If he falls in love, suddenly he has more energy than a person who lives on health food and exercises daily. What is the source and mechanism for this enormous flow of energy? How can we harness it and use it at will? These questions are especially important in the health fields because this energy is also the healing energy, or the life force itself.

A new definition helps make sense of this powerful but elusive and subtle energy: *Love is an attention or energy directed outward, the by-product of which is happiness. The opposite is need or desire, which is the same attention or energy directed back to the self, and the by-product of which is* un*happiness.* Reverse the direction of flow of attention or energy and you have the opposite feeling. Fall in love and you are in a state of bliss, but as soon as you want the other person to love you, you are miserable.

Fall in love and you have so much energy you can work day and night, but as soon as you reverse the direction of flow back to the self "Oh woe is me, aches and pains," you have so little energy you can hardly move.

Subliminally, we see this love energy. When a person falls in love, we say, "He's beaming, glowing, radiant, vibrant, turned on." Thus we see, at some level, an aura which brightens in proportion to the increase in love. Holy people or saintly individuals are those who approach total love, and they are depicted with bright auras or halos or surrounded by light. They also are known for their great joy, peace, and bliss.

Biblical accounts describe scores of such holy people who lived hundreds of years. This supports the concept that love energy is the life force itself or the healing energy. Need or desire, which is the exact opposite, roughly can be equated with what is called "sin," and we have read, "The wages of sin are death" or "Touch the forbidden fruit and you shall surely die." This is energy flowing in a direction opposite to the direction of flow of love energy or the life force. It is multidimensional and represents both physical and spiritual death. Anger is the most common emotion associated with heart attacks. Depression, which relates to need, not love, correlates with cancer. Stress, which is associated with worry, correlates with hypertension, diabetes, and ulcers. This list could go on and on.

Note: We do not find a similar list of medical ailments that correlate with feelings of love.

Profound truth often is profoundly simple once revealed. Perhaps this is so with our new definition of love. While this law that applies to the flow of love energy appears obvious, usually it remains a mystery throughout life. We start as little children, thinking that when we get what we want, then we will be happy. Wanting produces tension and a state of discomfort. When we get what we think we want, there is momentary relief of that tension and discomfort. This causes us to believe that satisfying our desire is the route to happiness. But soon we begin to want more, which propels us back into the state of discomfort and dissatisfaction. This wrong concept follows us throughout life. In Eastern disciplines, it is known as the Maya trap; and indeed, it is a trap because it snares many of us from birth to death.

O. Spurgeon English often spoke about how people always are trying to *get* something as a means of finding happiness. He described how little children think that when they are big, then they will be happy. When they get candy, then they will be happy. When they start school, then they will be happy. When they get a bicycle, then they will be happy. When they graduate, then they will be happy. When they get a car, then they will be happy. When they find a girlfriend or a boyfriend, then they will be happy. Next, it is when they get into college, then they will be happy. When they graduate, then they will be happy. When they get a job, then they will be happy. When they get married, then they will be happy. When they have children, then they will be happy; when the children are grown and leave home, then they will be happy; when they retire, then they will be happy. Finally they retire, and in six months, they are so bored they go back to work.

Sadly, many never learn that you cannot *get* happiness; it is the by-product of giving. We have all heard that it is better to give than to receive, but we lose sight of this almost as soon as we hear it.

Some have everything *but* happiness while others have *nothing* but happiness. Who has more? Our formula might dictate that the easiest way to become a saint, and enjoy greater peace and happiness, is to care and do for those who have nothing to give in return. By eliminating the possibility of worldly reward, we eliminate the thought and therefore the desire to receive anything in return.

Witness Mother Teresa helping the dying in the streets of Calcutta. They had little or nothing to give in return. While appreciation always is welcome, it is probable she did not even seek that. If appreciation were her goal, she might never have reached such heights.

Having does not preclude happiness, but attachment does. Avoiding ownership removes the possibility of attachment to objects, but there can still be attachment to rituals and even man-made religious practices that are not from scripture.

The closer we approach total love directed outward, with no energy moving back to the self, the brighter our auras become. This is in keeping with the words I heard during the night, "The aura is the edge of the soul." It makes sense that this is so. When we love, we are more like holy people, and our auras brighten. Could this explain the concept of drawing energy from the soul? Love provides energy. When we do something for someone else, which is love, we are more likely to succeed. Athletes sometimes perform beyond their capabilities by dedicating an event to a deceased teammate or to a child dying of cancer. Many mothers conquer life-threatening conditions because they have a child who needs them.

It is only when we approach total love, with no attachment to anything, that we approach the incredible fountain-of-youth vision I was given one night, in which a holy man appeared, from whom flowed a beautiful fountain of love energy, depicted as light and extending arm's length from the body from above the head and flowing downward. This love energy is the life force itself, which likely accounts for the extreme longevity among many of the persons in the Bible from millennia past, and for the longevity anticipated by Christians during the thousand-year period following Christ's return when total peace and love are to prevail.

<u>Scientific Versus Spiritual Analysis of the Flow of Love Energy</u>

When I began the study of love energy, I approached it like other physical laws. I searched for energy that follows precise unchanging patterns that are qualitative and quantitative and which are subject to precise measurement.

I found no such study related to the laws of flow of love energy in scientific investigation. Perhaps I did not search deeply enough in the scientific literature; but to the best of my knowledge, this has not been scientifically studied and quantified.

An odd thing did begin to happen, however. I began to receive information during the night regarding this mysterious energy, and that information proved to have validity. Later I discovered it matched what is found in Scriptures and is regarded as unchanging truth.

For this reason, this chapter on love energy necessarily contains more biblical references than references to anything in the known scientific world.

It is my hope that this will stir the interest of scientists. Science is open exploration, and the findings regarding love point in the direction of the existence of precise physical laws that are qualitative and quantitative. It also is my hope that the biblical references do not cause some readers to negate the important findings regarding origin and mechanisms, treatment and prevention of serious mental and emotional disorders. Similarly, it is hoped that reference to teachings related to one religious discipline do not cause persons of another faith to negate the total content of this book.

With this as a disclaimer, let us continue this exploration together.

When I programmed the dream to learn what to do to enhance spiritual growth, the answer was that I had to achieve total forgiveness and be slow to anger. That dream was followed by four weeks filled with the most outrageous situations I ever encountered. Coincidence? I doubt it. We are forever being taught.

It is hard to imagine the harm caused by bitterness, resentment, and nonforgiveness. Christ said it is just as great a sin to have the thought as it is to commit the act. Can you imagine how much of our life force is lost by holding on to angry thoughts? Many healers claim it is impossible to heal without first achieving forgiveness of others.

This translates into only love energy directed outward. If you express a certain amount of love, and an equal amount of anger/bitterness/non-forgiveness, what is your net outflow? How does that benefit you? How much positive energy are you accumulating? How bright is your aura? How lasting is your fountain of youth? How secure is your soul? Loving means reaching out to all people—not just to family. Christ noted that even the tax collector can do that, and therefore it is not to our credit.

We often hear it said that we must love the self first. This has great popular appeal and people are quick to endorse it, but it is the wrong direction of flow of love energy. Whenever I hear a preacher utter those words, I quickly retort with "Yes, and love God second." It takes a while before they can collect their thoughts and reflect on this. It is true that we should not hold anger toward ourselves, along with self-blame and self-condemnation. When we distinguish between the flesh and the spirit, then like Paul, we can identify with the higher calling and disparage the needs of the flesh. When we make that distinction, then we can dislike our wrong actions and wrong thoughts because we identify with and cherish the Spirit within.

Love your neighbor as yourself probably means *do* for your neighbor as you would do for yourself.

So the positive love energy may go out, but if it is directed back to the the self it is need or desire, not love. Negative energy must not be sent out, but may a person receive the pain and suffering of others? I learned of one discipline where persons picture sending love and healing to the whole world with each outward breath and receiving the pain and suffering of the world with each inward breath. Before jumping to the conclusion that this is a sick concept, do we not know someone else who reportedly took on all the ills of the world, all the sin and all the sickness and suffering of mankind for all time? And did He not say we must follow Him? Give love, and receive the suffering of others. Is this what Mother Theresa did? Through her loving kindness, she took their suffering and their grief.

This formula is like the laws of physics. If there is equal energy going in two opposite directions at once, nothing is accomplished. There is no positive net outflow of energy for our fountain of youth. Notice that now practically the whole world is moving in opposite directions. Like creates like. Love creates love. Hatred creates more hatred. Bombs create more and bigger bombs. Where is the endpoint? We read in Psalms: "A soft answer turns away wrath, but grievous words stir up anger," And in Proverbs we find "By long forbearance and calmness of spirit a judge or ruler is persuaded, and soft speech breaks down the most bonelike resistance."

Along with the fountain-of-youth vision was the awareness that this same fountain is available to flow through anyone. From ancient times, there are tales of persons searching the far corners of the earth for this elusive fountain of youth, never realizing it flows from within each person, as long as he or she loves with no regard for anything in return.

Simultaneous with this awareness was the realization that as soon as you *want* to live forever, you shut off the flow—because wanting to live forever is energy flowing in the opposite direction. You can want to teach forever or to serve forever, but as soon as you want to live forever, your attention or energy moves back to the self.

There is yet another dimension to this love energy.

Love and hate are not opposite sides of the same coin. It is love and need (desire) that are opposite sides of the same coin. When these needs are not met to our satisfaction, we respond by sending out negative energy: anger, hurt, bitterness, rage, even murderous impulses, and nonforgiveness that some of us cling to for the rest of our lives.

This is negative energy sent outward, which mathematically is equivalent to neutralizing an equal amount of outward flow of positive love energy.

Can you imagine the *net* outflow of love energy in a person who holds an equal amount of bitterness, resentment, and nonforgiveness? Much of this stems from very early in life when needs are great and everything seems unfair. This can rest deep in our unconscious minds, but as we practice methods of increasing our love by continually aiming our love and appreciation outward, even deep-seated unconscious bitterness will begin to change.

This same principle is stated in Proverbs 13:14: "The law of the wise is a fountain of life to those who depart from the snares of death."

This is akin to the commandment: "Thou shalt love the Lord thy God with all thy heart, and with all thy mind, and with all thy soul." This is the fountain of life—as long as you depart from negative energy flowing outward (rage, bitterness, nonforgiveness) and depart from desires of the flesh, for the self. These two are "the snares of death."

As the enlightened holy man instructed many years ago in answer to my question of how to become total love toward all people all the time: "When you want to hit a target with an arrow, aim only at the bull's eye." He meant to direct the love toward God. This allows for a much greater flow of love. When we love a person, we do not reach out as fully because we reach out with our own love-need combination, and the need portion of that continuum can be hurt. But when we reach toward God, there is no rejection and we cannot be hurt, so we reach more fully. Furthermore, we actually begin to emulate total love itself.

This is repeated in Proverbs 14:27: "Reverence for the Lord is a fountain of life to those who turn away from the snares of death." Jeremiah also refers to the Lord as *the fountain of living waters.*

In order to achieve this total love, this total flow of living waters, we must turn from harmful thoughts and deeds and from self-love and self-aggrandizement. We know that a family or a nation divided will fall. What about a mind divided between love and desire, or energy going both directions at once? Persons with power have their energy moving in one direction. Regardless of differences in beliefs, the commandment mentioned above is a scientific formula for all energy to move in one direction. It is a formula for maximum power and it is found in major religions.

The above references pertain to love, and love produces both happiness and good health. These considerations are particularly important in terms of treating physical, mental, and emotional illness. Physical problems heal faster when persons predominantly love, and mental and emotional illnesses can quickly disappear with love.

I recall an elderly nurse at a healing crusade who prayed, "Meet their needs, Lord. I am too old to bother with. Take care of them." Instantly she was healed of a severe back injury of many years duration.

From study of this love energy, it appears as though we benefit from loving and serving, with no regard for receiving something in return. Gifts are welcome, but if we do something for the purpose of getting something in return, that is not love.

In summary, the love must flow outward—but without desire, lust, greed for the self—and we must not send out bitterness, resentment, and nonforgiveness. But when we love, we receive some of the burden of those who suffer.

Two Separate Channels for the Flow of Energy

If we pair the inward and outward flow of energy differently, we gain still another insight and perhaps the most important of all: On one plane there is the sending out of love and the receiving of the suffering of others. On the other plane, there is desire and wanting things for the self, which includes lust and greed, and then sending out bitterness, hatred, and nonforgiveness when we do not receive what we want.

Love can be neutralized by an equal amount of pride, selfishness, greed, desire directed back to the self, or by an equal amount of bitterness, resentment and nonforgiveness directed out to the other person.

This different way of categorizing the flow of these subtle energies did not become apparent until I studied Romans 8. It is very powerful and I read it many times because I sensed it was of great importance. In Romans 8:2 we are told that the law of the Spirit of life has made us free from the law of sin and death.

It clarifies further that the law of the Spirit of life is in the Lord (God is love), and the law of sin and death is in the flesh. Nearly all 39 versus refer to one or the other of these channels, or the *result* of adhering to one or the other. In fact, this could be a common denominator for the entire Bible.

Thus, the love flowing through us is Spirit. We send this out to others and receive their suffering. We lighten their burden as did Jesus, the "man of many sorrows." We love so much, and the love brings happiness; but when we see the suffering of those we love, this causes sorrow and we receive their suffering. This is the God-channel. The other channel is strictly that of the flesh—with all its desire, lust and greed, causing hatred, resentment, and nonforgiveness.

<u>How to Increase Love Energy</u>

Prayer, meditation, and devotion will increase love energy. This can begin gradually, perhaps a few minutes every morning and every evening; and then as you begin to experience the benefits, you will begin to look forward to this and find more time for it throughout the day. Some are able to remain in a continuous state of devotion and prayer. These are very special people, and we automatically gravitate toward them, especially when we learn to recognize the love that flows through them. God *is* love, and when we focus on Him, His love begins to flow through us.

As you practice this, you might begin to feel some of that love toward all people, even toward those you have never met. This is a strange phenomenon when it first starts to happen. You see a person you have never met, perhaps just passing by in the supermarket or in the post office, and you immediately feel love toward that person. Is it the God within them you are seeing and loving or the Spirit that has increased within you which is doing the loving? You also begin to feel more love and compassion for those you have never seen or met.

The more love you express and feel during meditation and prayer, the more love that will begin to flow through you. You gradually become aware that you are a conduit for love. Spiritual experiences increase, including awareness of coincidences and synchronicities, voices and visions during the night—all of which cause you to feel more love and more appreciation. Once all service is dedicated to the Lord, or to helping others with no regard for the self, then new capabilities emerge and persons begin to accomplish what otherwise would seem impossible. When the Spirit takes over, things begin to happen; and as you experience this, you begin to recognize it more in others.

One time during meditation, I began thinking it was nice experiencing such peace and joy during meditation, but what happens when we get back into the real world? I thought of someone who owed me money and moved across the country. Later that day, the holy man with whom I was studying stopped by my dwelling with a book from thousands of years ago and opened it to the page. He simply said, "I thought you might be interested in this." To paraphrase what was written, it said that when we encounter injustices, we should take corrective action but not allow ourselves to be a benefactor of that action. In other words, we should take appropriate legal measures to correct a wrong, but donate any proceeds to charity. What a remarkable answer! We do the right thing, but are not part of it. We take correct action to bring criminals to justice. If we see a hit-and-run accident and we get the license plate number, we report it. Since we seek no monetary gain, we are free from attachment and we hold no malice.

This is totally consistent with the flow of love energy. We do what is right but eliminate any motive of personal gain. There is deep wisdom in this writing. In response to my question about everyday life not having the same peace as found in meditation, this holy man simply noted: "Like the banks of a river, gradually the entire river shifts."

He further suggested meditating for short periods of time throughout each day, one day each week, one weekend per month, and one long retreat each year until we reach the same depths of meditation during the brief intervals as we do during the longer ones.

Utilizing Love Energy in Therapy

Deeper understanding of love brings forth new therapeutic applications. This includes the recognition that love can be transferred through voice alone.

It is said that anxiety is contagious, and persons nearby become restless. The same holds true for depression. One person can cast a shadow over an entire room. Similarly, peace, joy, and serenity are contagious. They can be transferred from one person to another, but rarely do we encounter a person who exists in total love.

Fortunately, this love, peace, and tranquility can be transferred through a recording of a holy person; and this has a powerful impact on the listener. It is critical that the person listens with eyes closed. This shuts out as much as 75 percent of external stimuli and eliminates a large portion of internal stimuli as well, so the person is listening with far greater attention. The recordings serve as an infusion of love, which neutralizes both anxiety and depression. Some of the recordings proved more effective in twenty minutes of listening than two months of antidepressant medication.

Through greater understanding of love energy and applying it in our own daily lives, we can sort through each thought, word, feeling, action, and put it on the scale to determine love versus need. By "need," I mean desire. This is most useful in psychotherapy. If a person is miserable, it is because of wanting something. If a husband or wife complains bitterly about the spouse, this has *nothing* to do with loving the other person, it has only to do with caring about the self and wanting more for the self.

One man, for example, was agonizing over a lady friend who left him. I quickly pointed out that his agony related only to his need for her. If he truly loved her, he might be happy for her that she was doing what pleased her the most. So it was not a great love he was losing, it was a great need. When he recognized that it was need instead of love, he was able to relinquish it without pain.

Enhancing the love energy of a patient is an effective means of increasing the healing process. This holds true for both psychological and physical healing. Nonforgiveness is negative energy directed outward, which is the opposite of love. Without forgiveness, it is impossible to achieve the same level of love or the same degree of healing.

Patients who are injured or who have serious physical illnesses often are focused on themselves and their infirmities. This is the wrong direction of flow of energy, and it neutralizes their flow of love, their life force, their healing energy.

Depressed persons also are focused on the self, and this is the opposite of being in love or loving someone else. This is counterproductive when trying to heal. Two of the criteria for major depression are (1) loss of energy and (2) no interest in anything (anhedonia). With your current understanding of love energy, the reason for these symptoms should now be obvious: if the flow of the life force is reversed, this neutralizes energy and withdraws interest from the outside world.

Anxiety often accompanies depression and in fact it *produces* depression. This, too, is understandable through utilizing what you know about the flow of our life force. Fear and anxiety relate to conscious and unconscious worries about "what's going to happen to me?" This is energy moving inward which produces unhappiness and depression. This is the opposite of love, the opposite of energy directed out to others. This is why tranquilizing agents reduce depression. They reduce fear and anxiety, and this reduces the amount of attention and energy focused back to the self. Alcohol is not included as a tranquilizing agent for this purpose because it is the most powerful of all depressants. It also can produce terrible insomnia.

After many years of trying to unravel the mysteries of this invisible love energy and in trying to compare the outward versus the inward flow of positive energy and the outward versus inward flow of negative energy, I realize these are precise laws of physics that govern the outcome and that they are qualitative and quantitative.

O. Spurgeon English once noted that, as a general rule, people are capable of accepting only as much as they can give. Have you noticed persons who have difficulty accepting a gift or a dinner invitation? Compare their ability to give, to the same ability in those who have no problem at all accepting anything you offer. The more we are able to give, the more we are able to accept the gifts of others.

This formula applies in still another way. When parents truly have not withheld love from their children, the children are delighted to help them in their old age. They give back with joy. When such was not the case, when children were not treated with love, the children might feel they *ought* to help their parents in their old age; but for them, it is a monumental task because deep down they resent doing anything for the parent. They were not taught to love through loving example, and their unconscious minds have an awareness of this imbalance. This is why some delight in helping parents while others struggle and do so out of a sense of guilt. In this way the deeds of the parent are passed on from generation to generation.

For happiness and spiritual development, the children still must forgive and develop their own ability to love, even though they did not receive the same. It is critically important to learn to look beyond our own feelings that were hurt by others and reach out to help even the very ones who hurt us. Some might say, *especially* those who have hurt us.

Forgiveness

At first, I did not appreciate the magnitude of forgiveness of sins, reasoning that I have been a good person and have not done much that I considered wrong. On the scale of the average individual, that might be true; but when we add up all the negative thoughts, the bitterness, resentment, and nonforgiveness—some of which is deeply embedded and present since very early childhood—and we add up all the desires, self-aggrandizements, lustful thoughts, and greed, we begin to see that possibly very few of us ever move beyond the break even point for a positive net outflow of love energy.

Christians believe that with salvation, *all* is forgiven and forgotten. When we consider the sum total of all bitter, revengeful, spiteful, nonforgiving thoughts (negative energy outward), combined with all ego needs, desires, selfishness (energy we direct back to the self) over the course of an entire lifetime, that's quite a promise.

While the laws of physics, described above, seem easy to understand (once revealed), and while they are confirmed repeatedly throughout Scriptures, seldom are they recognized or applied in the field of mental health.

Treating patients through the understanding of love can cure both depression and anxiety. A person who achieves total love can neither be depressed nor anxious. I use a multidimensional approach to the treatment of depression, but the one factor I never lose sight of is the direction of flow of love energy. I always point out when the problem is primarily the patient's need, desire, or lack of forgiveness. This same enhancement of love energy is very valuable in treating psychosis because psychosis relates to a partial return to infancy with all the needs of the infant. When a person becomes predominantly loving, this is movement away from the needs of infancy and movement back into adult mind/brain/reality.

This also holds true for the addictions. At an addictions' unit, a counselor voiced the opinion that it is very important to show the patients that the counselor really cares about them. He was corrected and told it is much more important that he get the patients to care about him and to do something for him. He then recognized that he himself had overcome his own addiction when he began helping others with theirs.

Enhancement of love energy should be a part of every physical remedy because it is a vital ingredient to healing. If persons are angry or hateful, they will not heal as quickly or as well. There are numerous studies that demonstrate the enhancement of the immune system with love energy or prayer, but these studies are just touching the surface or catching a tiny aspect of this energy. A thorough understanding of the laws of physics, which govern this energy, is important because it enables us to identify the direction of flow of this energy and reverse it at will if it is flowing the wrong direction.

<u>Apathy and How to Reverse It</u>

Relationships that lead to marriage usually begin with intense love and romance. This is so wonderful that persons begin to want more, but as soon as they want more, it is gone because you cannot *get* happiness. It is the by-product of giving.

When people begin to want more, it becomes like shopping in the supermarket. Soon they want more for less, and the relationship becomes need oriented. Each begins demanding more and giving less. Eventually the needs of one or the other are hurt, causing one to pull away, and then we have distance and apathy.

Thus the energy shifts from moving outward to moving inward to not going anywhere, as the relationship moves from love to need to apathy. These three stages are equivalent to moving from hot to cold to lukewarm.

There is a formula for returning this to intense romance once more. That formula is to trigger the need, *but prevent all hurt and jealous feelings.*

This can be applied to the relationship that has become need oriented or even distant and apathetic. Here, one of the pair must make a move in the direction of independence, *but without causing hurt or jealous feelings.* It is important to stir only interest which is attention directed out from the apathetic one. This attention directed outward becomes love *as long as hurt and jealous feelings are not triggered.*

For example, one couple had been married for forty years, and the wife decided that was long enough. She had collected a shopping list of everything she found wrong in the marriage, and she decided to move out. Both believed strongly in one marriage, and neither would go against wedding vows or have an affair, so that was not a worry on the part of either. Nonetheless, the husband was quite upset about the separation.

This man really enjoyed dancing, so I suggested that he ask his estranged wife if she would mind if he joined a dance club, a group of people who went to different places throughout each week just to socialize and dance. He really didn't need her permission because she already chose to leave him, but it was critical for him to get her to say it was OK because her giving permission reduces or eliminates jealousy and anger on her part. He explained to her how he was getting lonely for human companionship, and she agreed to his pursuing his new interest.

Since she agreed to the arrangement, she could not justifiably feel hurt, jealous, or angry. Frequently, he invited her to come along. He was very loving and gregarious, and at the dances, he made certain none of the women were left out. If any lady had not had not been asked to dance, he would be sure to ask her.

One evening, his wife finally agreed to go with him to a dance. She watched in amazement as one woman after another asked him for a dance, and several told her how lucky she was to have him for a husband.

Her interest in him soon returned. That was many years ago, and today, they are living together as a very happily married couple.

This approach was learned partly through a dream, in regard to a very challenging therapeutic situation that was about to lead to divorce. In the mid-1970s, during sleep, I received information that the situation would resolve because it would prove what was written in the Gita, in terms of the three *gunas*: *sattva, rajas,* and *tamas. Sattva* is the highest level, followed by *rajas,* and then *tamas.* I equate *sattva* with love, or energy flowing outward; *rajas* with need or desire, or energy flowing back to the self; and *tamas* with apathy, or no energy going anywhere. There are biblical references to this as well. Christ made reference to preferring persons hot or cold, but definitely, not lukewarm. *Tamas* is the lowest of the three *gunas.* I equate it to apathy or being lukewarm.

In the Gita, it states that the route from *tamas* to *sattva sometimes* is through *rajas,* or stated in English, the route from apathy to love sometimes is through need. I realized then that it is possible to instantly convert persons from apathy to love by triggering need *but preventing hurt or jealous feelings.* It is possible to take the most distant, apathetic relationship—trigger need *but prevent hurt or jealous feeling*—and thereby precipitate intense feelings of love and romance.

Perhaps this is the formula the Lord uses in the book of Revelations and several places in the Old Testament. When people see utter devastation and carnage, terrors beyond imagination, they become fearful of losing their lives (need) and then turn their attention to God (energy directed outward); and as they think about Him, their need begins to turn to love and appreciation.

This treatment modality requires much more explanation than we have space for in this book, but it has saved many marriages that were destined to fail.

One more example is a sixty-year-old librarian who was married to a man who belonged to half a dozen organizations and was president of several of them. She could go to the meetings with him, but she felt ignored and left out of his life altogether. I suggested she become more independent, go places and do things on her own; but she would have to let him know she really cared about him, that he was number 1 in her life, and she preferred to be with him. There are a lot of social clubs such as dance clubs, bird-watching groups, book clubs, etc.; and she could ask if he would mind if she joined one of them. I told her to preface any question with "do you mind if . . ." and this would stir interest, but should not provoke jealousy. I also suggested she think about this for a couple of weeks and put it into her own words.

The very next morning, as he was hiding behind the newspaper and drinking a cup of coffee, she said, "Bill, would you mind if I had an affair?" He spilled his coffee all down his front, but the very next week he took her for a tropical vacation in the Bahamas.

Had she said "You don't pay any attention to me, so I am going to have an affair," she would have stirred hurt, jealousy, and anger instead; and the result would have been just the opposite.

This is not a recommendation for risqué behavior. This extreme example is used to illustrate this elusive flow of love energy; and the powerful dynamic of how to take the lukewarm person, trigger the need, *but prevent hurt or jealous feelings* and thereby propel the person into powerful feelings of love. Any movement toward independence can serve the same purpose.

Sigmund Freud, in *The Ego and the Id*, wrote that the effectiveness of the therapy of the future might depend primarily on the mobilization of energy. This mobilizes energy.

When you understand the flow of love energy, you can actually redirect it. To help a person recover from a serious illness, get that person to help someone else or to help others with the same illness. One of my patients with AIDS experienced a substantial improvement in his condition when he started counseling people in the hospital dying from the disease. Get the patient's energy flowing outward, have the patient help others, and encourage the person's spiritual practices. Here you might have to redirect the person from the "give me, give me, give me" prayers to "I love you, I love you, I love you" type prayer.

Fear is the antithesis of love, and it is counterproductive. It focuses attention and energy on the self. Picturing the self to be well, the body free from disease, knowing and trusting this is so, and helping others recover—perhaps from similar problems—is far more productive. For the healing process, it is important to avoid hatred, bitterness, nonforgiveness, worry—and to focus instead on intensifying love, caring, and doing for others with no regard for anything in return. Maximum enhancement comes through the expression of devotional love and appreciation. All of this increases the life force, the healing energy, and the recovery process.

With further inspection, this love energy continues to follow precise laws that are like other laws of physics and which are quantitative. Of all things to study in medicine today, it is the analysis of love energy itself which might be the most rewarding and productive. It is this love energy to which I hope to devote a large portion of the remainder of my life. Likely, it is the most important factor for healing and for longevity since Hans Selye discovered stress, and it is equally as invisible as was stress at the beginning of the twentieth century.

As an addendum since first writing about love energy, there is a growing awareness of the absolute importance of aiming for the bull's eye and directing love toward God. This truly enhances the flow of love energy because we do not hold back out of fear of rejection. We begin to emulate love at its source, and we begin to experience a multiplicity of blessings, which magnifies our love still further. The great commandment—to love God with all our heart, all our mind and all our soul—is a commandment of mercy and compassion, for nothing instills more joy and more blessings.

Chapter 19

Programmed Dreams

Enlightenment, in some ways, is similar to turning on a light in a dark room, enabling you to see things that otherwise were invisible. It is much deeper than that, however. It is a sudden, clear illumination of that which might have been out of our range of knowledge and experience for as long as we have lived.

Without a greater awakening, it is easy for a person to reject anything beyond the five senses as relating to imagination or fabrication. This book describes a number of accidental occurrences, synchronicities, and visions seen or words heard during the night. Some of these are remarkable in the insights and guidance they provide. Still, this differs from a person who truly is enlightened and is able to draw from a far greater knowledge than we ever thought possible.

To be able to achieve a state of enlightenment in which we can arrive at such revelations could require more years than are available in our lifetime. I personally have known only a few who have reached such levels.

The good news is that you do not have to be a yogi and meditate for fifty years in a cave to achieve enlightenment. When you fall asleep, you reach just as deep a level of consciousness, but you are unaware and do not know how to make use of this.

There are two effective techniques for achieving answers during sleep: The first is to decide to have a dream about a problem and decide that the interpretation of the dream will tell you how to solve the problem. Then further decide to awaken at the very *end* of the dream, remember it, and write it down.

The second technique is to decide your mind will work on a particular problem throughout all the altered states of consciousness during sleep, and when you awaken, your very first thought will be the answer.

Elmer Green, the grandfather of biofeedback, is a highly enlightened man for whom I have great esteem. We first met at Menningers in 1964. Throughout the years, our paths have crossed several times; and in the early 1990s, I told him about the programmed dreams and the miracles that occur repeatedly using this approach. I was honored when later he wrote in *The Ozawkie Book of the Dead* that what we achieve with the dream technique matches what they do with theta brain wave training. Theta training is useful for deep meditation. The remarkable thing about a programmed dream is that it requires virtually no training. Practically anyone can do it any night at will.

We will start first with examples so you will begin to grasp the magnitude of what programmed dreams enable us to do, and then we will elaborate on techniques.

For nearly four decades, I have found the programmed dream to be one of the most effective tools for finding solutions to problems. All patients, friends, and relatives were encouraged to apply this technique; and the results have been amazing. Answers often go beyond the person's knowledge and even reach beyond the dreamer to other people. Typically, a person with a problem thinks only of two or three solutions to the problem, but the programmed dream seems to search all answers and arrives at the very best one. When a patient says, "I'll think about that," my reply usually is "What do you mean '*think* about it?' Thoughts are irrelevant! You only can think of a few solutions when there are unlimited possibilities in the universe, and you can know the very best one any night at will. Get the enlightened answer!"

<u>Dreams that Reach beyond the Dreamer</u>

Recently, a woman programmed a dream to find a job. The dream was about housekeeping at the Marriott Hotel. She boarded a bus that morning, met an old friend who asked her what she was doing, and she told her about deciding to work in housecleaning for a hotel. Her friend replied, "Girl, this is your lucky day! I am supervisor of housekeeping at the Marriott, and I am looking to fill three positions." Coincidence? Perhaps, but Philadelphia is a large city. What is the probability of two persons riding the same bus at the same time and both thinking about the same job, in the same hotel, on the same morning after the programmed dream that told one to get a housekeeping job at the Marriott? How often should such coincidences occur? There is a point where it might be more reasonable to suspect a power outside of our realm of awareness operating to make the connection.

Another woman lamented that she wanted to teach school but did not have enough credits to get the certificate she needed, so she programmed a dream what to do. The next morning, she did not remember the dream; but while taking a walk in a neighborhood where she had not been, she saw an old friend of her mother and introduced herself. The lady invited her in for tea and said to her, "You'll never guess what I do. I'm teaching school. I didn't have enough college credits to get the certificate, so I am teaching in the Catholic school system where it is not required." Again, what brought them together to provide the very answer she asked for prior to falling asleep?

It is written: "Ask and you shall receive." This did not specify any particular denomination or even a spiritual belief. Indeed, all my patients, friends, relatives—over the course of thirty-nine years—have received enlightened answers when they programmed dreams. The amazing results, one after another, year after year, inspired me to search for the source of this enlightened information. Is it from within ourselves? Is it some external source? What about when you do not even program to have a dream and you simply are given information during sleep?

One night during a dream, I was explaining to someone how *easy* it would be to prove his theories. He didn't seem to understand right away, and I thought he must be a little simple. When I awakened, I realized *I* was the simple one to whom some *higher* self was trying to explain a research survey that easily would confirm or negate my findings. In the dream, it also was *me* doing the explaining, so are there two of me? One who produces revelations during sleep and the other who is slower to catch on? Is this what is meant by the Soul (?) or Self versus self? I suspect theologians will have the answers to these questions. I am just puzzled.

It is written that God wants everyone to come to know Him. Since everyone is unique, spiritual awakening must begin through a variety of means. Even answers to programmed dreams sometimes come in a dramatic way that moves the particular dreamer to take correct action. Later you will read of a young lady who followed my recommendation and programmed a dream to tell what would be the best thing to do about her pregnancy. She had been considering an abortion. Her dream was tailored to have the greatest impact on *her*, and after the dream, she would never consider abortion. So perhaps, *other* encounters of a spiritual kind are tailored to have the greatest impact on the particular individual.

My own journey began with meditation and consciousness training courses, and only later did I begin having experiences such as being told the name "Christina" for my younger daughter, Jesus appearing during sleep to answer my question about Him, and more recently receiving the incredible vision of the Trinity ring. For me these experiences were very real. This is something you might explore for yourself with a programmed dream. When you begin programming dreams and experiencing the validity of the answers you receive, you will gain confidence and trust in them.

The research design in the dream that I (my higher Self) was explaining to someone (who turned out to be me), was simple yet profound. Prior to October 1929, we had the gay twenties. People were prospering and gaining great wealth. Then in October, the stock market suddenly dropped nearly 50 percent. Persons were 70 percent margined, and many lost everything. Fear arose as to whether they would lose their homes or would be able to feed their families. Immediately 25 percent lost their jobs. People were jumping off rooftops as fortunes were lost overnight. The multitudes were devastated, and emotionally, the attention of mothers shifted away from their babies and focused on personal loss and survival.

Since the origin of psychosis is prior to twenty-four months, the research design was to take any complete sample of schizophrenic patients for one full year decades later—from any state mental hospital where birth dates were recorded—and compare the number with psychosis who were zero to twenty-four months old in October 1929 to those who were twenty-four to forty-eight months old. The study could be fine-tuned to compare the symptoms and diagnostic categories of those who were 23 months old, 22 months old, 21 months old, etc. during the month of October 1929. This tabulation could identify a peak age-of-origin and age range-of-origin for each symptom and diagnostic category related to infant separation trauma, and it could be accomplished in a very short period of time. It easily would confirm or negate our findings, and when controlled for other confounding factors, it would be even more significant.

The informative words during the night continued. Another time when I was struggling to write this book, during sleep I heard the words: "Bugs in the bones, use the mind of Einstein." In essence, it was saying, "The brain has limitations; use the higher mind." This puzzled me somewhat. Usually the words are precise, but this was like the person speaking did not have full command of the language. I couldn't even understand it at first. Was this in the form of some kind of parable, to be understood only in the spirit? Or was the particular messenger not as adept with the English language?

Who is this higher mind? Is it the same for everyone? None of my friends, relatives, or patients, in thirty-nine years received answers that I thought were wrong. I know there are negative thoughts that influence persons when they sleep, but when we program for the best answer, that is what we get. If it is true that we can know by the fruit, then this certainly indicates the answers come from a good source; and repeatedly, this has been independent of the person's belief system. The results are equal. So it doesn't matter what you believe. My experience—from interpreting on the average at least five dreams a week and sometimes ten or more over the course of thirty-nine years—is that the result does not depend on what you believe. When you ask for the best answer to a problem, that is what you will get. You might have difficulty interpreting it and you might not remember the dream, but we have ways around these obstacles.

If the answers come from a heavenly source and are given to anyone who asks for the best answer, then are we all brothers and sisters with one Heavenly Father? Christians and Jews await the Messiah. Could He be the same? Even Chidananda, one of the great spiritual leaders of India, often said to me, "Many names and many forms, but one God." You can find the answer for yourself any night at will. Just decide to have a dream about the Messiah and decide that the interpretation of the dream will tell you the truth about Him and exactly who He is. Then decide to awaken at the very end of the dream, remember it, and write it down. Many will have a personal visit.

Answers to Medical Problems

For medical problems, it does not matter if the answer is known in the medical field or not. For example, thirty years ago, I had an excruciating gall bladder attack, and the procedure at the time was to surgically remove the gall bladder. This time I used a different technique to get the answer during sleep. I decided my mind would work throughout sleep on the problem, and when I awakened, my first thought would be exactly what to do.

The first thought was the law of gravity applied to gallstones for the first time in modern medicine. The first thought was to sleep on the left side instead of the right. The gall bladder lies under the liver and points to the left. If one sleeps on the right side, any sand or grit goes to the bottom, and no matter how much it contracts, it stays there. But if you sleep on the left side, any sediment goes to the neck of the gall bladder, and with the first contraction, it is expelled.

Before fully awakening, I had the afterthought, "What happens if there are stones too large to pass through the bile duct?" Immediately the answer was, "Simply have the stones removed," with the implication, "because you never can form another."

I know who posed the thought. *Who provided the answer?*

The next night, I slept on the left side, and the problem disappeared. Five years later, it returned and I realized I was sleeping on the right side again. I corrected this, and the problem disappeared once more.

For years afterward, whenever patients mentioned gall bladder problems, I would ask in what position they slept. Eight out of eight who slept on their side slept on their right side. Statistically, that is one chance in 256 by chance alone.

A Jewish patient told me this was right out of the *Laws of the Halacha*, the ancient Jewish law from AD 200 to 300. Volume II, chapter 71, Order of the Night states, "It is strictly forbidden to sleep prone or supine; you must always sleep on your side, and you should start out sleeping on your left side."

On another occasion, there was something in my left eye. It became progressively more painful toward evening, yet I could not see anything in the eye. So I used meditation to discern what it was. I decided that the moment I reached the meditation level, the first thought would be the answer. A minute or two later, I heard the word "metal."

That sounded serious. I decided to have a dream about the eye, and the interpretation of the dream would tell me exactly what was in it and exactly what to do. About half an hour after falling asleep, I saw myself sharpening the lawnmower that morning. Then I had the thought, "It must be a speck of stone from the grinding wheel." Immediately came the answer, "No, stone would not have enough carrying power."

In a deep state of hypnosis, one might remember sharpening the lawnmower, but would not compare the specific gravity of a speck of stone to the specific gravity of a speck of metal and realize the metal is twice as heavy and would have twice as much penetration power.

Once more, I know who posed the thought. *Who provided the answer?*

The next morning, an ophthalmologist removed two pieces of metal from over my left pupil and said if I hadn't come in, they would have rusted and impaired my vision.

These last two examples were cited only because of the immediate answers to questions pondered while still partly in the dream state and the matter of *who* answered my questions. The examples themselves are relatively unremarkable compared to the dreams of my patients.

Complex Medical Problems Solved in Dreams

One patient in the mental hospital suddenly developed excruciating chest and abdominal pain. The internal medicine specialist thought it might be either a heart attack or a kidney infection, and he suggested transferring her to a medical facility. After persuading him to wait until morning, I told the lady—who was a good dreamer—to have a dream that would tell her what it was, where it was, how she got it, why she got it, and what to do about it.

She also programmed that I would be able to interpret the dream for her. You can program that you will be able to interpret your own dream, and then you will have only dreams that you will be able to interpret. In this case, she programmed that I would be able to interpret her dream. Oddly enough, I immediately knew the interpretation even though it was highly complex. I consider it possible that the immediate understanding was because of her programming.

In her dream, she and her husband were driving along a winding road where they should not have gone. Then in the dream, it began to snow. The snow got deeper and deeper, the car veered off the road, and it was covered over with snow. Just beyond where the car went off the road, the road came to a dead end and went into another road at right angles, and then into another road at right angles, and then into another road at right angles. To me, this was an anatomical road map of the intestinal tract with an obstruction at the ileocecal junction. But I didn't tell her this. Instead I asked if she would please draw the road map for me. She did, and it even was in correct proportion! The winding road corresponded to the small intestine and the dead end was the cecum. The first right angle was the small intestine entering the ascending colon, leading to a right angle at the transverse colon, and then to another right angle for the descending colon.

As soon as the car was covered over with snow, her husband said, "I have to cut off the engine." The first thing one does for an intestinal obstruction is shut off the fuel supply (the food intake). Then five or ten people came from the city to dig them out. Five or ten in dreams represents the fingers on two hands, and I did not know if this meant laying on of hands or surgery. When they were dug out, she and her husband were OK, but the three teenage children were gone. They were the reason for the obstruction. She wanted more of her husband's attention for herself.

Intestinal obstruction is an acute surgical emergency, so I immediately transferred her to a surgical hospital. But before she left, I warned her, "You better have a dream that will get you over this problem, otherwise they will be cutting you open."

At the surgical hospital, the diagnosis was confirmed based on the X-ray finding of fluid levels in the gut and blood electrolyte studies. Surgery was scheduled, and she took a nap to program the dream how to get over the problem.

In the dream, she saw a tall dark man wearing a turban—like from the Punjab section of Northern India—and he was massaging her abdomen. When she awakened, the obstruction was gone!

To the nondream programmer, for a lady to identify an intestinal obstruction in a one-inch segment out of twenty-three feet of intestinal tract—and then program a dream that gets rid of it—must sound like something out of *Alice in Wonderland*. But I am only reporting data and not attempting to draw conclusions for the reader.

I further learned that ten and twenty years earlier, a surgeon had operated on this lady for intestinal obstructions. I called the surgeon and asked where in the intestinal tract were the obstructions. He answered, "In the distal portion of the ileum." (Note: The ileocecal junction is the distal most part of the ileum.)

While others believed the prior operations caused adhesions, which then caused the obstruction, I noted that I had seen her neurotic needs increasing for at least two months, which is why I had hospitalized her. I hypothesized that more likely, she had learned to produce the obstruction and did so whenever there was a psychological need. The snow, incidentally, immediately struck me as representing dairy products that caused bloating and facilitated in some way the production of the obstruction. I had not asked her any of her associations to the dream, which is totally different from my psychoanalytic training. I instantly knew the interpretation perhaps because of her programming that I would. This is why I suspect the interpretation about the snow also is true.

Arthritis

In 1990, a patient began developing arthritis, and I told him to insist that his primary care physician refer him to a rheumatologist, which the doctor did. After six months, the arthritis was worse, so I told him it was time for a programmed dream. The next week, he called, quite excited. The arthritis already was getting better. The dream told him it was caused by stress, and the solution was long walks and hot baths. One week later, he no longer needed a cane.

This is not a solution one is likely to hear in medicine today. Commercial interests, ever seeking more profit, promote treating symptoms instead of addressing cause.

Transverse Myelitis

Another patient injured her neck at work and then developed pain and weakness in her left arm. Eventually, she also developed muscle atrophy there, along with pain and weakness in the right arm and then pain in the left leg. Her physician told her that she had transverse myelitis, which is inflammation of the spinal cord. He told her the cause and the cure were unknown, but he gave her a brochure to read about it. The brochure listed quadriplegia as a possible outcome.

I told her to program a dream that would tell her *exactly* what caused it and *exactly* what to do about it. In the dream, she was sitting in the dentist's chair, and he was removing a large number of teeth. Then she made the astute observation that these were only the teeth with the fillings. I asked her what kind of fillings she had, and she said silver fillings, which of course are 50 percent mercury, a powerful neurotoxin.

This was an uneducated lady who was a high school dropout. How did her mind know that a powerful neurotoxin was being leached from those particular teeth and that the neurotoxin entered her bloodstream and caused an inflammation of the affected area of her spinal cord? After having the teeth removed, her symptoms disappeared.

Raynaud's Disease

With Raynaud's phenomenon, the blood supply, usually to the hands, suddenly is compromised, and the hands turn purple and black. This is very painful and debilitating. The medical cause is not yet known, but this presents no obstacle for the programmed dream.

The first patient followed my instructions and decided to have a dream that would tell her what caused her Raynaud's. In the dream, she was chasing the maid around the house, then out into the driveway, and then she was slamming the maid's head into the blacktop. Suddenly, the face of the maid changed to that of her younger sister. She recalled chasing her younger sister around, as a child, because her father seemed to favor the younger sister.

This put her adult mind in great conflict with her child mind because as an adult, she loved her younger sister. Both the child and the adult mind and brain are hardwired to the rest of the body however, so when the unconscious rage of the child wanted to harm the sister whom the adult loved, the adult part of her mind shut off the blood supply as a means of blocking the violent impulses!

The mind is fully capable of doing this. Yogis have trained their minds to be able to direct the flow of blood. Elmer Green, in testing Swami Rama, found he was able to produce a ten-degree temperature gradient from one edge of his hand to the other and then reverse it at will. Thus it is possible to consciously increase or decrease blood supply to areas of the body. This supports the programmed dream finding that one portion of the mind can decide to cut off the blood supply to prevent an objectionable action by another portion of the mind.

One case does not prove a theory, even though I have not known programmed dreams to be wrong. Soon the next person with Raynaud's phenomenon appeared, and we were about to program the question once more. This was a devout Episcopalian nun, who was extremely gifted, but who was troubled by unwanted physical desires that tempted her. The programmed dream again elucidated the same duality: one part of her mind was vehemently opposed to the desires of another part of her mind, so it stopped her by cutting off circulation.

Both dreams showed an extreme need on one part of the mind to control an extremely objectionable impulse belonging to another part of the mind. With the first person, it was an aggressive impulse; and with the second, it was a sexual impulse that was thwarted by shutting off the blood supply.

More recently, a social worker brought a patient to the office with Raynaud's disease. I explained the origin of Raynaud's according to the two dreams. The social worker chuckled. The patient's Raynaud's started after she was raped, and the Raynaud's was on the inner aspect of her thighs!

Allergic Reactions

One time I developed a severe sore throat that lasted nearly three weeks. Medically, this is considered cancer until proven otherwise. A dream was urgently needed, so I decided to have a dream that would tell me what was causing it and what to do.

The dream was a vision of red, tight, swollen cells, with simultaneous awareness that this was esophageal lining and that it was an allergic reaction to pepperoni.

How long might it have taken for an ear, nose and throat specialist to determine that I had an allergic reaction to pepperoni? I stopped the pepperoni and the problem disappeared. Two weeks later, I tried pepperoni and the sore throat returned, confirming the diagnosis.

Another strange thing about the dream was the cellular detail. I probably saw esophageal lining while in medical school training, but I certainly would not recognize it thirty-five years later, and the highest resolution we had was a thousand power, which would have made the cells appear about the size of a pea. But in the dream the cells appeared nearly as large as a baseball!

This reminds me of the smallest subatomic particles being described by yogis thousands of years ago. The dream confirmed that such is possible and without requiring years of meditation and purification. The programmed dream can reveal similar levels of information the very first night. Purification still is needed for greater enlightenment and spiritual power, however, because power requires total forgiveness and control of angry thoughts so we do not bring harm to others and then back upon ourselves.

<u>Future Events</u>

Programmed dreams continue to amaze me. There seems to be no limit to what they can reveal. We demonstrated this repeatedly with cause and treatment for health problems that are not yet known in modern medicine. We also demonstrated it with dreams that reach beyond the dreamer more than can be explained by coincidence. This is similar, for example, to those facing hopeless situations and, then repeatedly beyond chance, finding that prayer works.

A number of programmed dreams have foretold future events with amazing accuracy. This does not mean that the dreamer will receive this particular miracle any night at will, but it indicates that such can happen and we should not exclude the possibility. In fact, *to exclude the possibility from consideration could eliminate the possibility for it to happen.* That would be like putting a problem into a computer and adding the stipulation that the computer cannot solve the problem.

One time a couple asked for advice about whether to get married, and I told them to program a dream. Furthermore, I said, it will be the same dream because there is only one best answer. I meant, of course, that it would be the same answer. Symbolism can vary. Both had the dream of being married, and the symbolism of each represented having four children. Many years later, after the fourth child was born, the woman required a tubal ligation because of complications in the pregnancy.

In another case, a man programmed a dream about starting a business venture with an Oriental couple. The people were honest, likeable, and hard working; but the dream told him the husband would have a heart attack and be unable to work, so he did not enter into the partnership. I do not know the outcome, but based on thousands of other program dreams, I would be surprised if this did not occur.

One of my own personal experiences involved an offer I had to purchase certain development property. On the surface, it looked like a promising investment. Crucial to the potential value of this property was the planned opening of a bridge across the bay. Persons were encouraged to buy two pieces of property because it would double in value when the bridge opened and they could sell the second to pay for the first. The programmed dream, however, revealed that property owners would all try to sell the second property at the same time when the bridge opened and prices would plummet. Essentially, that is what happened. Prices dropped, in some cases, by as much as 50 percent.

Information Beyond What Is Contained in the Mind

Information often goes beyond that which we would presume is contained in the mind. In fact, the programmed dream can provide knowledge that we know for certain was not within the scope of information available to us through direct, five-sensory perception.

For example, I once wrote a very strong letter to a patient who was taking too much Valium. Two nights later during sleep, I became aware that she was so infuriated by the letter she decided not to return. Then during sleep, I realized we both were at the same receptive level of consciousness, so I just pictured *her* deciding to come in the next day. When she arrived, she said to me, "When I got your letter yesterday, I was so peeved that I decided I would never come back. But when I woke up this morning, I changed my mind." She, of course, thought that *she* changed her mind when really all she did was read my mind. Anyone can do that during sleep, but few realize this.

Two patients with businesses saw their stores being robbed during a dream. The first saw someone cutting a hole in the roof of her pawnshop, lowering himself by a rope ladder and stealing guns. She called the police, and they told her they already caught him. He had set off the alarm. Another woman awakened with a dream that someone tied up her manager in the back room and was robbing her jewelry store. She called, and it had just happened.

When you program long enough for dreams, the mind becomes aware that you want to gather information during sleep, and it automatically does this for you. You might find yourself receiving important information you need to know. Sometimes the information can alert you to danger concerning a friend, and you will know exactly what to do.

One time, a dear friend, who I had not seen for two years, complained of a heart condition that kept recurring. He had dilation of the coronary arteries and then had a stent inserted, but still the problem continued. I explained programmed dreams, gave him a set of dream tapes to hear, and told him he would wake up with the answer. Two days later, he called from the University of Pennsylvania Hospital, saying the dream told him to "get it over with," so he went in for quadruple bypass surgery. I assured him the operation would be a success because I never knew a programmed dream to be wrong. I visited the next night, and he already had the surgery. That night, I received a clear message through a dream. He was up and running around, and suddenly one of the arteries burst. The words were "too soon." I knew this was a warning—not that it was going to happen, but that it would happen if he became active "too soon." I cancelled patients, went to see him, and explained the dream. It was just a warning not to get too active too soon. His son and wife were there and agreed completely that it would be just like him to be up and dancing the very next day.

I didn't program to have the dream or to awaken with it, but I was thankful for it. From my many dream experiences, I presume there are angels looking over us and protecting us, and they appear more often when we begin to program dreams. This is reflected in Psalm 16:7: "I praise you, Lord, for being my guide. Even in the darkest night, your teachings fill my mind."

Chronic Fatigue Syndrome

About twenty years ago, my brother developed chronic fatigue syndrome. After seeking medical attention, it became clear to him that physicians, generally, did not understand it at that time. So he began studying it himself. He has a photographic memory and has been known to read as many as ten books in one week. It didn't take him long to find out what had been written on the subject of chronic fatigue syndrome, but he still didn't know what caused *his* particular condition.

With some coaching, he programmed a dream that would tell him exactly what caused it and exactly what to do about it. In the dream, he was in a new office building with a contractor who builds offices. It was a large airy space with windows all around.

These simple details immediately made clear the cause and the cure for *his* chronic fatigue. One of the many causes of the disorder is sensitivity to mold and the neurotoxins they produce. There had been a fire at his office building. It was thoroughly drenched with water and began to grow *Stachybotrys*. That particular mold grows in ceiling tiles and is so toxic that it was considered for germ warfare. As a result of the dream, he relocated his office, and the condition improved.

Following Medical Advice Received During Sleep

As a note of caution, here are two examples of persons disregarding medical advice received during sleep:

The first person programmed a dream to tell him what to do about his back injury. He had been considering surgery. In the dream he saw himself after back surgery, and he was literally climbing the walls in agony. When I saw him next, three months later, I learned the surgeon had talked him into an operation, and now the pain was ten times worse. I was surprised that he didn't follow the advice from the dream, but reasoned there must be something he still could do. When he programmed what to do next, he awakened with a one-word answer. Sue.

The next case is tragic, and it pains me to even think about it. A dear friend's wife was diagnosed with breast cancer. Her programmed dream was of a woman who literally was cut in two—but she was still alive. Next she saw three beautiful young women in sheer negligee, but their feet were not touching the ground. To me, there was only one way to interpret this dream: Don't worry about disfigurement; at least you will still be alive—as opposed to finding yourself in the spirit world. Later that week I received confirmation through synchronicity. I walked into a postgraduate medicine classroom just as the professor was saying: "Integrative medicine treatment protocol number one for breast cancer is surgery."

I felt relieved that my friends knew what to do. Three months later I learned they had worked at the dream until they found another way to interpret it. Since the dream had told us what to do three months earlier, I could no longer be sure it had not metastasized. We all grieved deeply when she passed.

Moral Issues

For years, I had awaited the opportunity to try the programmed dream on a person who was thinking about abortion. In thirty-nine years, none of the dreams instructed anyone to do something morally wrong, so I was curious about the question of having an abortion.

Finally the opportunity presented itself. A young lady with a history of drug addiction became pregnant, and her mother was insisting she have an abortion. It was her first pregnancy. I told her to program a dream as to what to do about the pregnancy that would work out best. The next week, she reported the dream: she saw her two-year-old son lying dead on a cold steel slab in the morgue. She was still crying when she described her dream. The important thing is that after the dream, she was totally focused on saving her baby. She recalled seeing her father dead on a cold steel slab in the morgue, so this dream was designed specifically for her because the imagery is what would touch her heart the most.

Soon another opportunity arose. A patient's sister was thinking about an abortion. Immediately I wrote a dream to give to her that day: "I will have a dream *about* the pregnancy, and the interpretation of the dream will tell me *exactly* what to do that will work out best."

The next morning she wrapped her arms around him and was crying and crying. "What's the matter?" he asked. "I had the *dream!*" she shouted. "I was playing in the back yard with my baby, chasing it around the yard, rolling a ball back and forth to it, and pushing it in the swing." She continued to cry. For her it was an experience of total joy.

This dream does not involve telling the person what to believe or what to do. It comes from within the person's own soul. I like data, and I look forward to the first 100 of these dreams. But based on thirty-nine years of having all patients, relatives and family members program dreams, and never having a person receive a wrong answer, I would wager that it is unlikely a programmed dream will tell a woman to kill her unborn child. And, since the dreams are so powerful, few might be inclined to go against such a dream.

Wording is critically important. One must not program "What do I want to do?" That is irrelevant. It could be something quite foolish. The question must be "What will work out best?"

When the answer comes from within, it is from a higher source, and the person *knows* it is so.

Caution: Sometimes a dream will show a person doing the wrong thing, but will show the consequences thereof—that is, it will reveal, "If you do this, these are the consequences." For example, someone wanted me to partner in a business deal. I was not inclined to get involved in business, but I programmed a dream anyway. The dream was simple. I was sitting in a lounge chair, and it folded up with me in it. The symbolism was clear.

The Dream that Ended the Vietnam War

One of my dearest friends in life was Milton Friedman, not the economist, but President Ford's speechwriter. He was loved by everyone. When the Dalai Lama arrived in Washington DC, stepped out of his limo in front of the White House, looked out across the crowd of dignitaries and important people, he spotted Milton. It was like Milton was the only one he saw. Smiling broadly, he waved, and the first thing he said was "Hello, Milton!"

Milton was good friend of Edgar Cayce's grandson and had practiced Cayce's incubated dreams, which are like programmed dreams. Milton's sense of humor was unsurpassed, and this carried over into his dreams and speech writing. He loved to show contrast—not sarcasm, but contrast. I can still hear his words at the Council Grove meeting in Kansas, for example, as he deliberately drawled out the words: "We have a coalition of forty-four nations, three of which have armies." This of course was when President Bush was trying to gather support to apply pressure on Saddam Hussein.

Milton and I were planning to write a dream book together, which was to be called "Programmed Dreams and Incubated Dreams: From the Couch to the Whitehouse." His dreams would provide wisdom *with* humor. Every other page, people would laugh.

One incubated dream was of a more serious nature: Henry Kissinger had just given a speech saying we had to stay the course in Vietnam. This was aired on national television that evening. Milton was to write the speech for President Ford to present the next day, and he was supposed to show it to Kissinger first. Working into the night, he fell asleep and awakened at 3:00 a.m. with the words: "The war is over." This was pure wisdom derived through his incubation technique. He finished that speech, handed it to Ford in the morning, and apologized because there was no time to show it to Kissinger. "Never mind," said Ford. "This is exactly what I must say."

In telling the story, Milton was quick to add that it only ended the war *sooner*.

Dreams about Loss of a Loved One

So far, during the last twenty years, more than a hundred persons have ended terrible grief and suffering over loss of a loved one just by having one programmed dream.

Recently a young lady, referred by her father, had called her boyfriend on the phone. When he did not answer, she went to his apartment. There she found that he had hung himself. Had she been fifty years old, it would have been the end of the world to her; but she was only twenty, so it was far worse. For two weeks, she stayed at his gravesite, crying and praying.

For the first fifteen minutes, we utilized one of the power therapies to neutralize the horrible traumatic experience of finding him hanging in his apartment. The problem had been that each time she thought about the experience, she had to force it out of her mind because it was too painful. This could have continued for years. But with the trauma desensitization, she was able to bring it to the surface and neutralize it at the same time. The sudden relief she experienced astounded her. Before she left, I instructed her to have a dream *about* her boyfriend, decide the dream would not be upsetting, and decide the dream itself would resolve all upset feelings.

The next week, we spent a few minutes desensitizing any remnants of the trauma. We used the eye movement desensitization. With the first series of eye movements, she felt butterflies in her stomach. With the next series, she felt tingling in her fingertips; and with the third set of eye movements, she saw the butterflies flying away. The trauma was neutralized. That sequence took five minutes. Then I asked about the dream. It was one flash image of her boyfriend with huge angel wings coming out of his shoulders. Her greatest upset was because she is Catholic and feared he would not go to heaven as a consequence of the suicide. After the dream, she *knew* he was all right. Perhaps the sincere prayer, night and day for two weeks, made a difference. The dream provided knowing at a very deep level. She required no further treatment.

A fifty-year-old woman was grieving over the loss of her husband. She had never even dated another man. She had known him since she was fourteen, and she did not know what she would do without him. So I gave her the same instructions: "I will have a dream about Joe, the dream will not be upsetting, and the dream itself will resolve all upset feelings. I will awaken at the very end of the dream, remember it, and write it down."

The dream was the two of them getting ready to go out. He was rather slow, and it took him a long time to prepare himself. After two hours, the taxi arrived but still he was puttering. After another half hour, he managed to get into the cab; but after riding a few blocks, he said, "I left my wallet home," so they had to return for the money.

This is not uncommon for this type of dream. It is as though he were telling her—in answer to her question about what she ever would do without him—what on earth could she ever do *with* him! The dream did give her some peace of mind and a greater awareness that she might manage her time commitments better by herself and even manage other aspects of her life better without him.

In another case, a young man suddenly lost his wife in a terrible car crash. He was deeply in love with her and did not know how he could live without her. This was a very delicate matter, and it required lots of reassurance, but I gave him the same precise formula nonetheless. I told him to program a dream about her, decide the dream would not be upsetting, and decide the dream itself would resolve all upset feelings.

His wife had used credit cards recklessly, buying new clothes practically every day. In the dream, she told him, "Hey, you can open Suzie's Boutique!" This made it clear to him that death was not a terrible thing to her, and she was making light of it. The dream allowed him to gain another perspective on her death and helped him resolve his feelings of loss.

On another occasion, a bright-eyed young lady, who always was cheerful when she greeted me at the university, instead was crying and appeared deeply saddened. Her eyes were red and tearful as she told me that her eighty-year-old father had just been killed in an automobile accident.

I had only a few minutes between lectures, but I told her to program a dream about him, decide the dream would not be upsetting, and decide the dream itself would resolve all upset feelings. The very next morning, she was excited and even somewhat elated. She revealed that her father just jumped into the dream the same way he always surprised her. It was a very happy dream, and she knew he was OK.

Another woman was grieving over the death of her eighteen-year-old son. I instructed her how to have the programmed dream.

In the dream, he was twelve years old and was in some kind of a parade. He was smiling, looking happy, and was tossing rose petals to the spectators. She called out to him, but he did not respond. Then in the dream, she saw an uncle and a friend of hers—both of whom had died. They told her, "Leave him alone. Can't you see how happy he is?"

Later she programmed another dream to resolve all upset feelings. In that dream, her son ran up to his eight-year-old sister, picked her up, and carried her over to show her a rose bush. He looked very happy. After each dream, she felt better, knowing that her son was all right.

An elderly woman who had twelve children continued to grieve over the loss of four of them. She followed instructions and programmed a dream to resolve her upset feelings about their deaths. In the dream, she was at a wedding and all twelve of her children were there. It was a happy dream, and she enjoyed visiting with each one of them. She awakened feeling much better.

There is a variation of this dream which works for other devastating situations. Earlier this year a woman told me that her seventeen-year-old daughter was raped and the assailant then tried to kill her. Immediately I began writing a dream for her daughter to program: "I will have a dream *about* the rape. The dream will not be upsetting, and the dream itself will resolve *all* upset feelings."

The next month I asked the woman her daughter's dream. "Oh," she said, "my daughter confronted the rapist in her dream, beat him to a pulp, and woke up feeling good. She said this completely resolved the whole matter."

That's not the end of the story. Remember how the dream moves beyond the dreamer? The next day the rapist was caught in the process of raping another little girl and was severely punished.

Four Emergency Dreams

As I was leaving for California one morning, a former patient called from Georgia, crying hysterically, saying her husband had just died. He had spent all their money, the rent was due the next week, neither of their two vans were reliable enough to use, and she didn't know where she should live. I asked if she had paper and pencil. I had only a few minutes because I was in the line that was boarding the airplane. Quickly, I gave her four dreams to program: Decide (1) "I will have a dream about Fred, the dream will not be upsetting, and the dream itself will resolve all upset feelings." (2) "I will have a dream about where to live, and the interpretation of the dream will tell me the answer." (3) "I will have a dream about the two vehicles, and the interpretation of the dream will tell me exactly what to do." (4) "I will have a dream about the rent money and the interpretation of the dream will tell me exactly what to do."

I made certain that the wording was precise, and for some reason, I had unusual confidence she would get all four answers and solve everything.

I saw her a month later, and that is exactly what happened. In the dream about her husband, he realized that she loved him and she realized that he loved her. It was a very touching dream, and she felt good afterward. The next dream told her to move back to Philadelphia where she had friends and relatives. The dream about the vehicles told her to give one to her husband's daughter; and that the second one, with a minor repair, would get her to Philadelphia. The fourth dream told her to move before the rent was due.

Each of these problems had been monumental to her, yet they were solved in four nights with four dreams.

Spiritual Growth

The above are but a few of the many thousands of programmed dreams encountered over the years. Even a mere five dreams per week for the last four decades would be more than ten thousand; and I tell nearly all my patients, friends, and relatives to program dreams. Each one is remarkable. As long as the dream pertains to the question programmed, it will provide useful information.

Can you imagine the potential for developing spiritually through seeking the very best means of doing so during the dream state? The guidance automatically would be tailored to fit the requirements of each particular person.

The many years of programmed dreams confirms for me that when you program for the best answer, you do not get something unholy. You will not receive an answer to do something wrong. It is written: "Seek and ye shall find." This is a means of seeking and finding, and in my experience, what you find will be for the best good of all. Since the programmed dream answers provide the best course of action, if we follow them, how can we go wrong? Who can argue with the benefits of making the right choice at every juncture?

Those who have had years of experience with prayer or who have delved intensely into the realm of spiritual communication have come to trust in the answers they receive. Why? Perhaps it is because of the reliability of the results they receive, with ever increasing appreciation for those answers, and ever increasing love—which further enhances the connectivity to the source.

The same trust develops when you begin to program dreams for the best answer to a question or the best solution for a problem and repeatedly recognize the truth and goodness in what you receive.

In my own life, my first instruction to pray actually came through a programmed dream. During a time when my younger daughter was having great difficulties in her social life, I programmed a dream to find out what I should do. The answer was to pray, which surprised me because I had never prayed before. Thankfully, this turned out well.

The programmed dream can be used for seeking what to do next on your spiritual journey. The guidance is there, ready and waiting. Any time. For those who question who the Messiah is, simply program a dream and see what you get.

Not long after beginning to program for dreams, visitors began to appear during sleep. It was about thirty-five years later that I read in Job 33:23 that if we catch even one out of a thousand of the messages the angels are trying to convey, our lives will be blessed.

Somehow, once we begin to seek answers, messengers appear just to give instruction, show by example, provide advice, or help in various other ways. Sometimes we recognize immediately these are highly evolved spiritual beings. Other times, they appear as ordinary persons, and only as the dream progresses do we recognize a divine presence. On occasion, there is just a soft voice during sleep, which might be spoken with great compassion; or there can be the rare but formidable voice that awakens us from a sound sleep and keeps us on course or gives us important instructions.

I have never seen an angel with wings during sleep, just messengers—sometimes swift, sometimes as ordinary people who gradually reveal great wisdom, sometimes as yogis, especially in the years following my first journey to India. The spoken words—whether soft, gentile, compassionate, or the powerful, authoritative one—emanate from holiness; and you know to trust these words from the first time you hear them.

Those who would like to intensify their spiritual life can program to have a dream that will reveal exactly what to do. The possibilities are unlimited. In recent years, I have come to know a number of people who report they maintain a continuous dialogue with the Lord. These persons are particularly gifted in the spirit, but it is possible that even they could acquire additional information at this deeper level just as Daniel demonstrated so well with his night visions.

Recently, a religious lady challenged me with, "Everything we need is in the Bible, so why do we need to program dreams?" After hearing some of the remarkable dream answers to medical problems, she saw merit to programming dreams.

Techniques

It is important that you know *how* to program dreams. The clinical vignettes are to show you the magnitude of what you can do by using this technique. It is easy for you to learn. Then you can use this valuable technique and teach others to do it as well.

In logical sequence, let's start with how you prepare yourself the night of the dream. The first item to address is how to enhance your ability to even remember the dream. Here is a list of suggestions:

1. Freud slept on hard boards so he would not sleep too soundly, and this enabled him to remember dreams better. You can try that, but it is a little heroic in this day and age.
2. Try the magic dream pill instead: take 100 mg of Vitamin B-6 the night before and you might even have the dreams in vivid color. Or you might instead take Vitamin B-100, which has 100 mg each of Vitamin B-1, B-2, B-3, B-5, B-6, a trace of B-12, folate, and choline—all of which enhance memory. If this is not sufficient, you might add more of the vitamin B-6. I would not recommend going beyond 300 mg.

3. Meditation at bedtime is helpful. This enhances the ability for dream recall. It brings our awareness to a slower brain wave frequency, which might be why we have more awareness during the slower brain wave frequency of the dream state. This is just a guess as to why meditation at bedtime is helpful for dream recall, but experience verifies that it is helpful regardless of actual mechanism.
4. It is critical to decide in advance to awaken at the very *end* of the dream, not in the middle of the dream or between dreams. This is when you remember it best. All you have to do is decide that is when you will awaken, and you will. Have you ever tried to awaken at a certain hour in the morning and you awaken at the precise time? Most people refer to that as "setting your mental alarm clock." If the mind knows when the hands of the clock are precisely on the designated hour, it certainly must know when you come to the end of a dream.
5. Deciding in advance that you will remember the dream and that you will write it immediately are two more critical factors. The mind will do what you direct it to do. You must of course have paper and pencil right there; otherwise you negate the programming to write it immediately.

    You can even decide to awaken at the end of the fourth dream, remember it and write it down. We have four to five dreams every night, and if we awaken at the end of the fourth dream, we do not miss as much sleep. You can also decide to awaken at the end of each dream, begin writing, and then wait for the next. Each successive dream can add clarity and provide additional information.
6. Try to begin writing *before* you open your eyes. Place your left hand on the edge of the page and start at the little finger and go to the next and the next. When you open your eyes, you are no longer at the same state of consciousness, and it might be more difficult to remember the dream. Sometimes it is best to review the dream before you even move because shifting body position, in some people, can cause them to lose the dream.

One time, when having difficulty organizing a lecture on programmed dreams for a 1979 presentation in Buenos Aires, I decided to organize the whole thing during sleep and just start writing before opening my eyes. To my surprise, I outlined the entire presentation with eyes closed, and this became the basis for the 1981 programmed dream tapes.

In addition to the above six factors for remembering the dream, there are at least six more factors that influence your ability to even have the dream:

1. The intensity of the need to have the answer will have a bearing on result. If you are desperate for an answer, you are more likely to remember the dream. A person with cancer, for example, is more likely to get the answer as to what to do. Based on my experience, I personally trust that answer beyond anything known in medicine today.
2. Negative programming will prevent you from attaining an answer. If you decide in advance that you will not be able to do it, this definitely will interfere. It is like plugging a problem into a computer but adding the stipulation that the computer cannot solve the problem. Simply decide your mind will retrieve the answer, and then observe what you receive.
3. Your own resistance to receiving the answer can interfere. You might be afraid you will get a certain answer you do not want to hear.

    For example, a teenager who had a small inheritance decided he wanted to spend the entire amount on an expensive sports car. I told him to program a dream to tell him what to do. He tried night after night until we both realized that he was not getting the answer because he was afraid he might get an answer he did not want to hear. So we adjusted the programming to find the answer that would bring the greatest happiness. Now he no longer could have resistance to getting the answer because he could not object to having the greatest happiness. The answer came that same night, and it was to get the cheaper car. Once he received the answer, he had no resistance to it whatsoever! The answers bring us to a deeper level of knowing, and they tend to erase all doubt.

    Countering resistance to receiving an answer is an important consideration. Otherwise if we are afraid we will get an answer that we do not want to hear and would not want to follow, this can prevent us from having the dream.

    This dream technique is wonderful for teenagers. They can be very difficult to advise because in establishing their own independence, they must go counter to what the parent suggests. So just ask them to try the dream technique and offer to support whatever they get because it is highly unlikely there will be a wrong answer. When the teenager finds the answer during sleep, it comes from his or her own mind, which also eliminates resistance. Further, there is the absolute knowing that it is the right thing to do and that it will work out best.

4. When the dream is used to help others, there can be an enhanced ability to receive answers. Ego needs are less likely to be involved. This results in purer flow of love energy. When you are doing something for someone else, you really do enhance your performance. Chapter 18 on love energy explains this in more detail.

From what you know about dream programming so far, you should understand how Daniel was able to get his programmed dream to interpret King Nebuchadnezzar's dream even though Nebuchadnezzar refused to tell him the dream. We do not have the same boundaries or limitations of our abilities during sleep. We use the same programmed-dream technique he used: only he referred to his dream as a night vision. His vision was enhanced through love, prayer, agreement, fasting, faith, and necessity. Some people are more gifted than others. There are very few Daniels and very few Edgar Cayces, but nearly anyone can receive enlightened information during sleep.

5. Write the programmed question the night before. The language must be precise, and the question must be formulated with great care. The wording cannot be sloppy or inaccurate.

For example, one seventy-year-old lady wanted to travel to the Orient, but she was afraid of heights and was apprehensive that someone would book her in the tenth floor of a hotel somewhere in China, so she was hesitant to go. For weeks, I had her programming what to do about her fear of heights, and she kept having dreams of being in one-story buildings. Finally, somewhat disgruntled, she complained, "I don't seem to be getting the answer." I too was puzzled, but then during sleep, I realized she was getting the answer every single night. What should a seventy-year-old lady do about her fear of heights? She shouldn't go into tall buildings! When I told her this the next week, she was still disgruntled, but clarified, "I don't want to know what I should do *about* my fear of heights; I want to know what I should do to get *over* my fear of heights!" That was a different question. Her dream answer the following week was not psychoanalysis; it was every day one step higher.

Thus you can see the precision needed when formulating the question. The difference of a single word can result in an altogether different answer.
6. While the question must be formulated with very precise wording, it also must be all-inclusive. That is, we must not place limits on the answer. It would be foolish to ask "Should I do choice A or choice B?" because there might be a million alternatives, half of which might be better.

The programmed dream technique is perfect for research and for discovery. With direct access to the most creative levels of mind, and with access to information that goes beyond body/mind/brain/thought to total enlightenment, we have access to unlimited resources. It has been exceedingly valuable for identifying origin and mechanisms of mental and emotional disorders.

Many of the best insights came from the dreams of patients. One of the greatest insights into how the mind works in mental illness came from a patient who led a very useful and productive life as a professional, but she had one isolated and near-fatal flaw. If her husband came home late from work, she might slash her wrist. I made several interpretations that fell short of the mark. She knew that she became extremely upset because her alcoholic father often came home very late when she was a young child, but her knowing this did not help.

Finally, when the therapy was failing, I asked her to program a dream to tell us a new therapeutic technique that would help us get her over this problem sooner. In her dream, I was to make a tape recording of things that would upset her—she was to take the recording home, play it, and go berserk while recording her reaction on a second tape. Then in the dream, she was to bring the second tape into the office, play it, and then say, "Oh, how stupid!"

In other words, what we realized is that what is real to a person depends on the reality the person is experiencing at the time. When she was experiencing two-year-old reality, that was real until she no longer was in the two-year-old mind. In the dream, when she came to my office and was back in her adult mind, and then heard the recording of her two-year-old mind reacting to my tape, it sounded stupid to her adult mind.

After she had that one simple dream, any time she started to get upset about her husband coming home late from work, she would hear the little voice saying, "Oh, how stupid!" This immediately brought her out of the earlier reality every time.

It was her dream that showed me with greatest clarity that people shift to earlier realities. Any psychoanalyst knows that the interpretation must be made at the level the person is experiencing. The dream allowed her to cross-index the two realities when the adult was able to see what the infant was experiencing and realize that to the adult mind, it was stupid.

No matter what kind of medical or psychiatric problem the person has, the answer as to cause and what to do is available during the dream state. Not everyone receives it every time, but the information is available and your mind can do this. Formulate the question with precision, and decide you will receive the answer.

Many psychiatric problems are easy to solve during sleep. There are volumes written about the first dream brought into psychoanalysis because after a lengthy psychoanalysis, the analyst looks back and sometimes sees that everything was contained in the first dream, which really was a programmed dream.

The patient, on the night prior to beginning psychoanalysis, has his most intense desire to know what is in the unconscious mind and what caused it. That night, he has a dream that gives him the answer. If the analyst were aware of programmed dreams, he could tell the patient to have a dream the next night that would tell him how to get over his problem sooner. In some cases, this could save years of treatment. On occasion, the programmed dream technique has enabled persons to overcome deep-seated emotional problems in a single night.

One patient, for example, had extreme anxiety; so I suggested he have a dream that would tell him the origin and what do, and that the dream itself would solve the problem for him. The next day, I received a call from his wife, asking, "What on earth did you do in one hour to get him beyond twenty years of extreme anxiety?" The answer had to wait until the next week when he told me the dream. In the dream, he and his cousin were wearing Eaton suits (short pants with jacket and bow tie worn by little boys). In castration anxiety dreams, there is often a "spare." In this dream, it was his cousin.

In the dream, they were going down the escalator into a department store. Department store symbolizes Mother, with all the goodies inside. Then in the dream, a horrible monster started coming down the escalator, and he knew that the monster would kill him. He was terrified. But when he reached the lower level, he discovered that the monster was a friendly guy who just wanted to play and dance and have fun and who never would harm him.

Three years earlier, I had met with him a few times and told him about castration anxiety and what caused it; but without psychoanalyzing him, this interpretation missed the mark because the interpretation was at the adult level while the experience was at the level of the child. In the dream, however, he was the child; and when the child learned the father would not harm him, the adult no longer had anxiety. In essence, the dream provided a one-night cure.

Lastly, about programmed dreams, when you begin programming and do this with regularity, your mind comes to know that this is what you want it to do, and you will begin receiving guidance on a regular basis. Different things will begin to happen. You will awaken at the sound of the doorbell, which actually does not ring, but it serves to awaken you just as a powerful thought or important message is coming through. This can cause you to question whether there is some other force trying to tell you something and using the doorbell trick to make sure you wake up and remember it.

At times you will receive verbal messages that come through at the speed of thought and in which there is never an extra word. These messages are truly enlightened statements, and they cause you to wonder about the source. These occur without programming, but might relate to something of particular importance to you at the time.

Some people even report enlightened visitors, or visions, during the night which are most helpful. One patient who had a terrible problem with a twelve-year-old daughter, for example, solved that problem completely with her first programmed dream; but then an American Indian chief began visiting her during sleep. She had told me she wanted to be a writer.

I chuckled to myself because I thought her to be an unlikely writer, but then the Indian chief began providing deep, profound wisdom.

One night, she asked him how he became what he is. He described being a young lad, in a small village, who was very egotistical and constantly calling attention to himself. Eventually he fell in love with a young maiden, but she would not pay attention to him. So he thought if he became wealthy by their standards, then she would pay attention to him, but still she ignored him. Then one winter, there was not enough food; so he thought if he could go on a hunt and bring back some food, then she would pay attention to him.

Before venturing forth, he stopped at the dwelling of another family and found them all frozen to death. This touched him deeply and made a special impact on him.

On the hunt, he was about to kill a giant elk when by some freak accident, he was mortally wounded. In his dying moments, his only concern was about bringing food to the starving people in the village. In other words, there was no concern for himself, not even for his own life. In his dying moments, his need instantly became love, and that's his story of how he became what he is.

There are two Bible quotes that relate specifically to the Indian's story: The first is Jesus saying, "No man has greater love than he who lays down his life for a friend." The second relates to a parable given by Jesus to the effect that those workers who arrive at the end of the day get the same penny. The Indian had shown total love in his dying moments. *This is the Indian's story of how he became what he is.*

Even the expressions the Indian used were stone-age expressions, such as "The smallest man with the smallest stone can bring down the biggest redwood tree." Another expression was, "You have to walk down the mountain before you can climb the mountain."

It took fifteen years before I realized that the programmed dream probably is what most people describe as the miracle of prayer—only with a simple technique for receiving the miracle any night at will. If it helps, then decide that it is prayer, and then pray in this special way to get the answer to the riddles of your own life.

Chapter 20

Babies Need Mother's Love

At the core of this book is the fact that babies need mothers, and the *emphasis* has been on prevention of separation traumas, with delineation of illnesses caused by separation traumas at specific ages in the first thirty-four months of life.

But that is not the whole story. There are many other important factors in child development. *Mother's love and the quality of mothering* is critically important at all stages of development, particularly in the earliest years of life, and even during pregnancy.

While practically everyone *knows* that babies need mothers, careful scrutiny of the subtle but changing lifestyles in modern societies makes it clear that merely "knowing" that babies need mothers is not an adequate safeguard against the gradual shifting of importance of the mother's role in child rearing.

In recent decades, there has been an erosion of the importance of motherhood, brought about by commercial endeavors through nearly all news media. The impact of this global commercial endeavor might not be recognized for what it is. It results in a shift in societal values that can work against the *expression* of mothers' love, and even cause her to minimize the importance of spending time with her own child.

Mothers are being pulled from all directions to focus on different needs—needs of their own, needs to purchase goods, to have more, be more, do more, get more. They are coached on how to find the very best daycare center and the best babysitter. Having a career is made into an ideal, and then they are enticed into having the finest new car and wearing the latest fashion. Some surveys report that the average American adult watches approximately five hours of television per day with as much as one-third of some programs devoted to those powerful enticements known as commercials.

Thus the values of motherhood are constantly being eroded and challenged and replaced by the changing societal values and pressures to conform. The joy of motherhood is in danger of being lost as more of a mother's time is taken from her true love, the precious little bundle she loves so much. Consequently we have to shift our focus back to our babies and away from the distractions that abound all around us in our materialistic world.

In the wild, a mother bear watches over her cubs, and her attention is focused on protecting and feeding them. She is concerned about potential dangers to them; and her focus is on nurturing, guiding, teaching, and training them for the demands of their world to come. This is pure love, as demonstrated in a lower species. Is this still the primary focus of the highest species of all? Are our other needs artificially increased to a point where they begin to detract from our love? Are we bombarded with so many distractions and misleading temptations that our attention is taken away from what should be most important to us? Have we bought into "I need time for me" to the extent that the baby's need for a mother's love is not even recognized? The needs of the adult do not begin to compare with the needs of the infant.

These are questions and issues we must search in earnest, for we have seen that we cannot *get* happiness, it is the by-product of giving. And a new baby is a one-way street; it is total need into which we give our all. This is the real means of mothers achieving happiness, and it is the means by which mothers, through example, teach their babies how to love, so that they too might find happiness.

The remainder of this chapter is all about babies need for mothers' love.

Development of Love and Security Even Prior to Birth

Relatively little is known about emotional development prior to birth, but there is reason to suspect this occurs. It might, therefore, be a good idea for an expectant mom to begin thinking about the baby and visualize holding it and loving it before its arrival. Some mothers even read to their unborn babies and feel this helps them learn to read.

Dreams of patients I analyzed indicate awareness of external events prior to birth. Even an amoeba, a single-cell organism, can sense and react to danger. How much more developed is the human embryo? Science is open exploration, and the impact of extrauterine environment is yet to be determined, but the thoughts and emotions of the mother could play a major role.

There are many studies attempting to show that traumatic experiences in the second trimester of pregnancy have a high correlation with later development of serious mental disorders. These include death of father, poor nutrition, or starvation.

These are thought to cause an impact through nutritional and hormonal changes experienced by the infant. This could have some bearing on development, or it might even alarm the infant and serve as antecedent trauma that cause subsequent trauma to be experienced as more severe.

More likely the researchers are measuring the impact of separation traumas in the first two years of life and do not even suspect it: How secure is the mother who gives birth to a new baby after the father has died? Does she have to leave the baby to go to work? What about the mother who was starving during pregnancy? How secure is she about her food supply over the next two years? What are her living conditions? Does she have to struggle to provide food for the family?

Even though the second trimester traumas probably impact primarily on the mother-infant relationship during the next two years of life, the attitude of the mother toward the unborn baby must not be overlooked. We don't know the full impact this can have, but the comfort and security felt by the mother is important throughout the development of her child and could be important to its earliest development, its sense of security, and its sense of being wanted and loved. While this has not been measured and quantified, I would recommend that love for the baby should start even before conception.

<ins>Caring for the Baby at Time of Delivery</ins>

It is important to consider all factors surrounding the birth process. Natural childbirth education is important because it reduces the mother's fear, reduces pain, eliminates need for anesthesia, and facilitates delivery. During internship in 1962-1963, I delivered at least a dozen babies in one week, and perhaps as many as twenty. It was a brutal process, with episiotomies, anesthesia, using forceps, and stitching wounds. I was amazed at the improvement in technique when our children were born using methods taught in natural childbirth education. The trauma was markedly reduced. Now it appears to have shifted back the other direction. Approximately one-third of deliveries are with cesarean section. Why is this so? Does this interfere with mother's immediate attention to the baby?

Loving the baby includes preventing physical trauma. It is critical not to immediately clamp the cord because much of the oxygen supply still comes through the cord before the lungs are fully operational, and early clamping can cause petechial hemorrhages throughout the brain. This is demonstrated in animal studies. The practice of circumcision, without anesthesia and without the mother present to hold and comfort the baby, can be quite harmful. It serves as an antecedent trauma that can make subsequent traumas more severe, and it might be the reason for the greater incidence of autism in boys over girls.

It is also important that the baby be with the mother following delivery. Unless absolutely necessary, it should not be kept for hours or even weeks away from the mother in the hospital following delivery. If adoption is planned, nine months should be sufficient time to find an adoptive family. The lengthy delays required by adoption agencies to do their work is unacceptable. There is hard-data evidence that this causes as much as a tenfold increase in borderline personality disorders. Sadly, scarcely anyone has noticed.

In primitive cultures, babies are stroked for the first twenty-four hours following delivery. This brings consciousness to the surface, and some of these babies are able to jump up and run at just six months. If tape is placed across the abdomen of newborn kittens so the mother cat cannot lick the umbilicus, the kittens are much slower to learn to walk.

The First Three Years

Ideally, the mother needs help so she can spend plenty of time with the baby; and it is good for her to feel happy, relaxed, and secure. She must be free to enjoy the baby and delight in whatever it does. It is important to the baby that the mother enjoys their interaction. This causes the baby to know the mother values it, which provides added feelings of love and security.

The mother is the one person who can stimulate the baby's development more than anyone else. She is the one the baby wants and needs. Holding and feeding the baby provides a means for the transference of love. A friend once joked, "God was so serious about mother's love that he hung the milk on her chest." Certainly, the cradling of the baby in the mother's arms, holding it close to her heart, and caressing it in the feeding process provide a far greater opportunity for transference of love energy than placing it in a crib with a bottle.

It would be very difficult to replace the mother. The baby learns fundamental life skills, warmth, and caring through interaction with the mother. That is how the limbic system develops. The baby makes a sound or a gesture and the mother responds, then the baby replies and the mother does something more. The gestures and sounds of the mother are truly remarkable, and men would hardly be able to duplicate these. This is strictly right-brain activity.

Breastfeeding is a tender interaction between mother and infant in which the infant takes in part of the mother. Fortunately, it is not the only means of transferring love, but it is perhaps more important than we realize. In its growing love for the mother, the infant develops a wish to devour the mother, and often this coincides with starting to bite. This was noted in the section on eating disorders.

It is interesting to note that when Christians take the sacrament, following the instructions of Jesus, they break a piece of bread, which is to symbolize his body, and pour a cup of wine to symbolize his blood, and then they partake of these. This symbolizes ingesting part of Him as the infant does with the mother in developing *its* feelings of love. Could part of the reason for the sacrament be to help return the person to the love in the mother-infant feeding relationship? Does feeding also symbolize becoming one with the mother as the infant desires to take in the mother through engulfing her? Breast-feeding certainly brings a greater closeness between mother and infant. Christians are taught to be as a child and are taught He is in them and they are in Him. There is something of greater importance in this early relationship and early desire to have the mother within. It is so important that it has been given a place symbolically in worship in a major religion.

A hard glass bottle propped up in a crib cannot have the same effect as pressing against warm, soft tissue, being held and caressed, and taking in part of the mother. Feeding becomes just as much a part of the learning process as the sounds and gestures the two of them make, in harmonious rhythm, with love. One of the first times the baby learns to modify aggression through love is when it begins to bite. This is not learned through biting a rubber nipple.

Animal Model

Much can be learned from the animal kingdom. As I watched the deer in my woods one evening, soon after the bucks had shed their antlers, I saw one buck licking the wounds on the head of another; and this went on for at least ten minutes. It was done with great tenderness, and this was not long after they had engaged one another in fierce combat.

I surmised the one had been victorious—driven by instinct—and now was sorry for the pain he had inflicted. Afterward, the other reciprocated; but the feeling tone was a little different, and he only licked the other's wounds for about a minute. I sensed he had lost, but there was forgiveness and acknowledgement of the other's gesture nonetheless. They no longer were combatants. They renewed their bonds and were friends once more.

Survival in the wild depends on this life force called love. Telepathy has no language barrier, and they communicated perfectly well. We have lost much of this ability to communicate. In the horrific tsunami of 2004, for example, which killed 225,000 people in eleven countries, only the animals and the aborigines knew to get out of the way. They were more in touch with this life force from which most of us have departed. It is this life force called love—so tenderly displayed with forgiveness by the deer in my yard that day—which might be learned through the tenderness and caring communicated during breast-feeding.

Teaching the baby to love is one of the most important things the mother can do. The person who learns to love finds greater happiness, for happiness is the by-product of love.

Aiming for the Ideal

Whether the baby is breast-fed or not, it needs as much love and attention as it can get from the mother. Being a mother is a full-time position. The father and other family members should do all they can to support and help her. When the first baby is born, the mother suddenly finds herself immersed in a new twenty-four-hour-a-day responsibility. The baby's needs that were provided during the previous nine months do not suddenly disappear.

Life circumstances vary from family to family, economic and educational backgrounds are different, and a range of difficulties arises that require attention. In addition, some mothers are more stressed than others; some more worried, anxious or depressed; some have more needs of their own that must be met—and child-rearing practices vary from family to family. All these circumstantial differences impact the individual and contribute to variation from person to person. Nonetheless there still is the common denominator, in the patient, which is defined by the age at time of early separation trauma.

We can only aim for the ideal and do the best we can. Understanding the needs of the baby helps in our approach to the ideal. There is much individual variation, and some exceptional persons managed to provide adequately for the baby even during conditions of war.

Maintaining Love in Early Child Education

The first years of life are ones of rapid growth. They also represent a unique time for learning. Young children can learn to do things that adults never can do, such as instant math and perfect pitch. The mother can help the child learn these special abilities even though she can never attain them herself. Fathers gradually gain in importance to the young child and can assist in the learning process, but the emphasis should not be on the actual learning. This will occur quite naturally. The focus must be on *enjoying* the baby. This is showing love for the baby, and it is richly rewarded later in life.

Parents often try to teach a child by pointing out faults. This might be out of ego needs instead of love and a sincere interest in addressing the needs of the child. We can never improve on a person by tearing the person down. Children are very sensitive, and they cannot grow under such circumstances. While they need correcting, the emphasis must be on encouraging them, rewarding their love, and supporting their growth. Parents, because of their emotional ties with the children, are in a unique position to give the most valuable and enduring gift they can provide: love energy.

When we plant a flower, we make sure it gets the right amount of sunshine, the right amount of water. We might till the soil and add fertilizer, and then we clear weeds from around it. We might also prune it and direct the way it grows. Luther Burbank, the great botanist, also spoke loving words to his plants and asked them to do what he wished. Cleve Baxter, the polygraph expert, conducted remarkable studies of telepathy with plants and showed how they responded immediately to our thoughts. Plants do respond favorably to kind, loving words, and experiments repeatedly have demonstrated their dramatic response to prayer.

Certainly the child has as much sensitivity as a plant and can be nurtured in a similar way. Never underestimate the telepathic ability in a child. Try a guessing game with an eight-year-old, and see for yourself. They can read your thoughts.

I was aware of this and had trained both our children in telepathy. They could tell what I was thinking, but I couldn't tell what they were thinking. This proved to be fortuitous one time. My wife had lost a removable gemstone setting from her ring, and we searched all over for it for at least six hours. Finally our elder daughter who was four said, "I don't know why you are looking in the house. It is in the leaves next to the curb." We quickly drove to the nightclub where we dined the night before; and there where we had parked the car, in the leaves next to the curb, was the gemstone sparkling in the sun.

Still we could have done more. Early childhood is an ideal time to focus on spiritual growth and development, but I was unaware of spirituality myself. Children have unique abilities in this area, and these can be nurtured. I think of my new friends, Martha and Bob, who had their first spiritual encounters by age five and then grew to spiritual giants. I learned too late for my children to benefit from guidance in the area of spiritual experience. Like many parents, I too look back to reflect on what more I could have done.

In addition to accessing spiritual growth and development, perhaps the best guidance for child rearing is already written. If the child learns to live by the principles taught in scripture and does so because of inspiration from spiritual experiences, the child will have optimal preparation for life. Psalm 1 states clearly, "Blessed is he who delights in the laws of the Lord. He is like a tree planted next to rivers of water. He bears much fruit, does not wither, and prospers in all he does."

To successfully convey this to children, to instruct them to follow the path of love, and to teach them to recognize and tune into that which already is within, provides an opportunity for them to reach their full potential. This might be the greatest gift you can give your child.

Love them, nurture them, guide them through example, and let them grow.

Appendix

THE UNIFICATION MODEL FOR MENTAL ILLNESS
Clancy D. McKenzie, M.D.
© American Mental Health Assoc., 1998

ABSTRACT:

The author has identified a traumatic origin to serious mental/emotional disorders, which is confirmed through statistical analysis of survey data. A significant correlation is identified between separation traumas in the first two years of life and the later development of schizophrenia, and another significant correlation is identified between the identical traumas in the next year of life and the later development of nonpsychotic major depression.

The theory proposed is that of delayed Posttraumatic Stress Disorders from infancy: Separation trauma in the present precipitates a flashback to separation trauma in the first years of life, resulting in a partial awakening of the entire earlier gestalt—i.e., an awakening of the earlier mind/brain/reality/feelings/behavior/chemistry/physiology and neuroanatomic sites that were active at the earlier time.

This model accounts for biological change and allows for genetic predisposition. The voracity of the findings, however, indicates that infant separation traumas might be prerequisite for serious mental disorders to occur. This could have profound implications for prevention.

PREFACE:

While attention in recent decades has focused on biological change found in those suffering from schizophrenia and depression, new indications are that biological change might be the *result* of the disease process and not the cause.

If this is so, then biological research alone cannot identify all aspects of etiology, prevention, understanding, or insight psychotherapy. Biological findings are critical to the Unification Model, however, because they demonstrate the reactivation of earlier developmental brain structures, confirming that portion of the flashback experience.

To know where one's particular area of study fits into the overall structure, enhances one's ability to further that area of research. Like pieces of a puzzle, when one finally grasps where everything goes, the pieces fall into place more quickly.

THEORY:

Central to the Unification Model is the finding of delayed Posttraumatic Stress Disorders from infancy and the Two Trauma mechanism. Everyone understands when a car backfires next to a Vietnam Veteran and suddenly he begins speaking Vietnamese, grabs a gun and hides in the woods for a few days. A loud noise in the present precipitates the flashback to a loud noise in the distant past, and the veteran begins experiencing and behaving as he did at the earlier time. This is thought to occur because during combat the veteran's life was in extreme danger. The mechanism is so obvious that no one has conducted a comparative study to determine if noncombat individuals are affected by a loud noise in the same way.

What few realize is that more terrifying than war trauma to a soldier is separation from the mother to an infant. For 150 million years of patterning of the mammalian brain, separation from the mother has meant death. Thus the human infant is quick to misinterpret common events as threats of separation from its mother and therefore overwhelming threats to its survival. Then 10-20-30 years later, instead of a loud noise precipitating the flashback, it is a similar separation from some other "most important person" (husband, wife, girlfriend, boyfriend)—or group, which precipitates the *initial* step back in time.

The parallel concept, when transposed from the awakening of adult war trauma in the combat veteran to the awakening of infant trauma in the schizophrenic, is more difficult to grasp. Bullets and bombs are readily understood, but moving to a new house, or the birth of a sibling—even though potentially overwhelming to the infant—does not seem sufficiently traumatic to set the stage for the later flashback experience. Likewise, combat reality and behavior is easily recognized in the veteran, but infant reality and behavior is not as easily recognized in the adult schizophrenic.

It is puzzling why the reality and behavior of the schizophrenic is not more readily recognized as belonging to the infant. When one sees a full-grown man sitting in the middle of the floor screaming "Mommy!" "Mommy!" it seems obvious. The author first observed this as a small child in 1941. An 18-year-old girl was running nude through the lawn sprinkler in the front yard, squealing with delight. It took a quarter of a century to realize this was perfectly normal behavior, but transposed in time. Had she been 18 months old instead of 18 years old, no one would have thought anything odd about her behavior. With careful scrutiny virtually every piece of bizarre reality and behavior observed in the schizophrenic can be seen to mimic that of an infant—and with careful cumulative observation, correlating age of trauma during infancy with symptoms in the adult schizophrenic, it becomes apparent that the reality and behavior of the schizophrenic matches that of the infant at the time/age he or she was traumatized. After such cumulative study one begins to recognize a peak age and age range of origin for each symptom or disease category, and instead of *un*reality one begins to recognize that it is *earlier* reality the schizophrenic is experiencing (McKenzie, 1981, 1984, 1986; McKenzie and Wright, 1996).

Biological Change:

To expand the theory into the biological realm, let us first consider early brain development. The powerful mechanism of ontogeny recapitulating phylogeny does not stop suddenly after intrauterine development is complete. The infant progresses phylogenetically from earlier to later developmental structures, beginning with the reptilian and old mammalian portions of the brain, which are active from birth. At least a portion of the old mammalian brain must be active in order to have rutting, sucking and crying responses, but the Moro reflex and other survival mechanisms are present in reptilian brain. Critical pathways are accessed as one passes through earlier structures. Only after initial stages of development do the rudimentary higher cortical structures begin their massive growth. The language centers in the left posterior superior temporal gyrus, for example, begin their rapid growth spurt when the toddler enters its stage of rapid accumulation of new words and the ability to speak. Pearce (1977, 1985) describes a progression through age specific windows of learning, which begin in the first hours after birth. Some abilities that are not accessed during the narrow range of progression through the specific early structures cannot be learned later in life. Doman (1974, 1984) identifies which structures are active and developing at what ages, and demonstrates the unique ability of children to learn such things as instant math or perfect pitch at specific early ages and not later in life. With instant math a child less than two years old can instantly calculate lengthy math problems that adults are not capable of learning to solve mentally.

Thus when the schizophrenic flashes back and awakens a delayed Posttraumatic Stress Disorder condition, his flashback is biologically different from that of the combat veteran who flashes back to war experiences, because the schizophrenic returns to the phylogenetically earlier developmental brain structures he was progressing through while experiencing the extreme emotional distress that accompanies the separation response.

Kardiner (1941) coined the term physioneurosis to describe physiological remembering at the cellular level, in what now is called Posttraumatic Stress Disorder. Physiological remembering at the cellular level is particularly important in the schizophrenic process. The shift of activity to the earlier developmental brain structures, depending on when during infancy the person was traumatized, can account for activation of various regions of the brain that contain proportionately more of the neurotransmitters involved in the schizophrenic process. This includes reactivation of those structures that were active when the infant/toddler was overwhelmed and perhaps in a state of terror, and it includes reactivation of the chemical/physiological processes that were taking place then. Nemeroff (1993) demonstrates long-term reduced production of cortico stimulating factors in persons who experienced early separation from their mothers, and he views this as the cause of depression. According to research findings that will follow, separation traumas as experienced by the infant in the first two years of life correlate with the later development of schizophrenia, and the identical traumas in the next year of life correlate with the later development of nonpsychotic major depression. Paul MacLean, in personal correspondence regarding "The Anatomy and Psychodynamics of Psychosis" (McKenzie, 1984), agreed with the concepts and wrote: "It seems quite clear that the traumatic experiences in infancy and early childhood could set up a storm in those unstable structures of the phylogenetically old parts of the telencephalon that appear to be involved in the separation response. Somewhat analogous to an epileptogenic focus, the poorly dampened neural mechanisms would allow the storm to 'perseverate' or to be easily reactivated."

Neurotransmitters:

Earlier brain sites are reactivated as a result of the flashback to moments of extreme emotional distress. Along with the reactivation of earlier developmental sites there is an increase in levels of neurotransmitters produced there. This includes an increase in Dopamine (Breier), an elevation in CSF norepinephrine (van Kammen), changes in modulation of seratonin (Krystal) and a disruption in glutamatergic function along with an increased density of glutamate receptors (Mahlorta). Because of the reactivation of earlier portions of the mind and brain, it is not unreasonable to attribute the change in production of the neurotransmitters to the reactivation of the structures that were active at the earlier time. Change may occur as a direct result of reactivation of the structure producing the neurotransmitter, or it may occur indirectly—i.e., instead of learning perfect pitch or instant math, the infant/toddler—during a period of excruciating distress—may have learned how to produce the changes in neurotransmitters, and does so upon returning to the earlier gestalt later in life. The decrease in the CSF tridecapeptide Neurotensin (Nemeroff, 1994), for example, may be the result of such a process. Before drawing conclusions based on neurotransmitters alone, however, let us review other biological changes involved in the schizophrenic process and search for parallel findings.

Brain Atrophy:

In schizophrenia there is a shift of thought processes from those of the adult to those of the infant. Thus there is a relative deactivation of higher, rational thought processes, and a reactivation of feelings/ behavior/ reality belonging to the earlier time. Higher cognitive processes, memory encoding, language, speed of response, smooth eye pursuit—all were learned as the infant/toddler was progressing through developmental stages. When the schizophrenic shifts to earlier reality and behavior, functional deficits begin to appear—as well as atrophy of the brain structures responsible for the particular functions lost. Since the atrophy is associated with deactivation of the higher cortical structures, it is not unreasonable to attribute the atrophy to the partial disuse of those structures, as occurs in any other part of the body not being used.

Perhaps the clearest example of this is the massive development of the left posterior superior temporal gyrus at about the time when language development is at its peak. According to Crow (1990), the development is so extensive that the sulci elongate and the differences between the two hemispheres can be seen on gross examination of the brain or even on MRI. The schizophrenic shifts to a trauma that occurred prior to the peak age of development of language, and according to Crow, the left posterior superior temporal gyrus in the schizophrenic atrophies proportionately more than any other area of brain. This is simply a disuse atrophy. When the individual shifts activity to a region of brain, which was active prior to the development of a second region, that second region necessarily becomes less active and undergoes disuse atrophy.

LITERATURE SUPPORT FOR INFANT SEPARATION TRAUMA:

Before moving into the scientific proofs of the theory of traumatic origins of serious mental/emotional disorders, it is necessary to support the significance of infant trauma with references from the literature:

From the Posttraumatic Stress Disorder literature we learn that the younger the age at which the trauma is experienced the more severe the impact on the subject (Boros; Williams and Siegel; Kilpatrick; Hyman et al; Pynoos & Eth; Raifman; Zelikoff; van der Ploeg & Kleijn; Janet, 1919; Eth & Pynoos; Gampel, 1988, 1989; Kestenberg; Kestenberg and Brenner; Klein, 1974, 1983; van der Kolk, 1988; Spitz, 1945, 1975.) The infant is the youngest of all and therefore the most susceptible to trauma.

Paul MacLean (1973, 1985) identified separation from the mother as the most painful of all experiences to the mammalian infant, and MacLean's only means of eliminating the cry response was to surgically cut the connections between the old mammalian and the reptilian portions of the brain, effectively leaving the creature with the brain of a reptile.

Renee Spitz (1945) noted that in many institutions, in spite of the best of medical care, 50% of infants died if they had established a good relationship with the mother and then were separated prior to two years. Anna Freud (1953) noted that providing one constant mother figure for each group of infants, instead of a rotation of nurses, eliminated the infant deaths. Harlow (1958, 1979) noted that apes reared by a terry cloth mother would not mate, and one that did simply batted her infant away when it came to feed. Bruno

Bettelheim (1967,1968) attributed infantile autism to trauma during the first 18 months of life. Margaret Mahler (1979) identified trauma in the first 18 months of life as correlating with the later development of *childhood* schizophrenia, and considered the birth of a sibling to be very traumatic to many infants. Kraemer (1984) noted that monkeys separated from their mothers during infancy were more prone to alcoholism. Thus there are countless indications in the literature that infant traumas of separation from the mother are particularly stressful and lead to serious disorders.

LITERATURE DESCRIPTION OF DELAYED POSTTRAUMATIC STRESS DISORDERS:

The next area of literature search pertains to descriptions of delayed Posttraumatic Stress Disorder. Two of the best descriptions found were by van der Kolk and Ducey(1984,1989) and by Samuel (1990). Van der Kolk and Ducey described Rorschachs in "Mr. D." before and after the original traumas of ten years earlier were awakened: "Card after card reflected the same shift from earlier bland denial to later excruciating living of past horrors." Samuel described a combat veteran with three purple hearts, whose most terrifying experience was when his company accidentally disturbed a nest of hornets in the jungles of Vietnam. They were totally defenseless as hundreds of thousands attacked, and some men had hundreds of stingers embedded in their faces. This man functioned relatively well for 15 years after returning from Vietnam. He was married, had children and was gainfully employed. His life was a success until one day, at his place of employment, he found the ceiling of the men's room covered with hornets. His life suddenly became a living nightmare as he no longer was able to work, sleep or function. This is a clear example of the delayed type Posttraumatic Stress Disorder, and it is the same mechanism found for schizophrenia and other serious mental/emotional disorders.

The development of the delayed Posttraumatic Stress Disorder in the unconscious mind prior to its awakening as a full blown syndrome is similar to the concept of isolated core nuclei of consciousness (Janet, 1886) and the concept of unconscious fantasies from early childhood that later surface as the neuroses in the adult (Freud, 1926).

In schizophrenia, once the original trauma is awakened by a major loss, separation or rejection in the present, the infant and the adult exist side by side. With all serious mental disorders, after the initial reaction is precipitated by a known psychosocial stressor, recurrences can occur with little or no additional stress. According to the former *DSM III*, once a Major Depression is precipitated by a known psychosocial stressor, subsequent episodes can occur without apparent further provocation. Similarly, alcoholism—once awakened—is reawakened with but one drink. Following an acute phobic reaction the individual has a phobia. The same holds true for anxiety attacks, panic disorders, schizophrenia and more. Thus it appears that the initial activation of an earlier core nucleus of consciousness paves the way for reactivation with little or no provocation—and it appears that this same mechanism operates in most, if not all, serious mental/emotional disorders.

SCIENTIFIC STUDIES:

It has been relatively easy to prove that separation trauma is a primary causative factor in the later development of serious mental/emotional disorders. Future studies, to identify the peak age and age range of origin for each symptom/diagnostic category, and to determine the relative risk factor for each trauma at each age, will be far more involved—but necessary for prevention.

Researchers can begin with any trauma that causes the infant to feel threatened in its relation with its mother. The infant can feel threatened by common everyday events, such as the mother or the infant being hospitalized, the family moving to a new house, or the parents separating or divorcing. Some of the traumatic experiences are not suitable for study, however, because it is not possible to date precisely when the baby felt traumatized. Divorce, for example, can be preceded by months of disharmony, any time during which the baby can experience traumatic emotional separation.

One trauma proved ideal for study, however, because the precise date it occurred was known and recorded, and because it was traumatic to many infants. This was the birth of a sibling. In generations past, women remained five days in the hospital following delivery, producing significant trauma.

All studies conducted by the author were of patients born in this country, born in a generation *prior* to the advent of the working mother, and *prior* to managed health care—which forces mothers to leave the hospital the same day or the day after delivery. For purposes of study, this may have been fortuitous: Separation is more traumatic after good bonding has taken place in the first 4 to 6 months (Spitz, 1945), and many mothers now are working prior to this bonding taking place. The one day versus the five-day hospital stay is far less traumatic to the older sibling at home.

In the first study (1981) 60 patients who were schizophrenic and who were living in group homes were polled to determine how many had a sibling <18 months younger. An equal number of super normals, who had full affect and were leading useful, productive lives, were asked the same. Of the 120 subjects, 20 had siblings < 18 months younger. Of the 20, 3 were from the super normal group and 17 from the schizophrenic group. Using the binomial theorem, this reached the .001 level of significance. The research design was endorsed by John deCani, Chairman of the Department of Statistics at U. of Pennsylvania's Wharton Business School.

A modification of that design was applied in 1994, and the first 35 middle aged to elderly schizophrenics with one sibling less than 3 years younger were polled to see how many had a sibling 1-2 years younger versus how many had a sibling 2-3 years younger. The preponderance was so great in the 1-2 year younger category that again the .001 level was achieved with the first 35 patients. The identical study was conducted using 35 nonpsychotic major depression patients, and this time the preponderance was so great in the 2-3 year younger category that the .001 level of significance was achieved with the first 35 patients. And by mixing schizophrenic and depressed individuals and doing the same study—looking for mutual exclusivity (i.e., schizophrenia and major depression with psychotic features in the 1-2 years younger category, and Major Depression without psychotic features in the 2-3 years younger category)—the .001 level of significance again was reached with the first 35 patients.

Hearing voices was found to have its origin in emotional trauma prior to 24 months, i.e., prior to the age of origin of non psychotic Major Depression. In a study of 50 persons with very severe Major Depression, 15 had siblings born prior to 3 years, and of the 15, 7 heard voices and 8 did not. Hearing voices versus not hearing voices lined up with having a sibling before or after 24 months, in 14 of the 15 cases—again reaching well beyond the .001 level of statistical significance.

These findings should not be surprising because we know the language centers develop primarily after 24 months, and when the patient shifts to the brain cells used prior to that time he develops the language dysfunction of hearing voices. We already considered the fact that in schizophrenia when the person returns to the area of mind and brain that was active prior to the massive development of the language centers, that region of brain—which becomes less active—undergoes an atrophy which we attribute to disuse.

For those who require larger studies, Sarnoff Mednick was kind enough to test the birth of a sibling trauma on the 6,000 patients in the Finnish data base on schizophrenia and confirmed the author's findings for this particular trauma. The .001 can be achieved using groups of much smaller size, however.

Future studies will reduce or eliminate most genetic, familial and environmental factors, because siblings of the schizophrenics will be used as control groups. The findings related to broad age ranges can be narrowed to the identification of the peak age and age range of origin for each symptom/diagnostic category related to infant traumas—and if not related to infant traumas the same research design reveals that as well.

DATA FROM MAY, 1997 APA MEETINGS:

Having gained an overview of the concepts, let us see how they might apply to biological and neuropsychological schizophrenia research findings. For a current cross section of research findings we will first review those presented at the 1997 APA Meetings in San Diego, omitting but a few because of redundancy:

Several of the presentations pertained to response time in schizophrenia: Parwani et al described an impaired central inhibitory mechanism in response to the acoustic startle response as measured by pre pulse inhibition; Hazlett et al found the same and attributed it to frontal lobe dysfunction because PET, coregistered with MRI, indicated lower rGMR in the superior, middle and inferior frontal gyrus bilaterally, which was proportionate to decreased pre pulse inhibition; Willis-Shore et al—while not finding a correlation with I.Q. or frontal lobe dysfunction, found a slower reaction time in schizophrenia as measured by lexical decision tasks which was proportionate to conceptual disorganization and suspiciousness. These findings would be consistent with a shift to earlier structures and a return to less mature levels of function.

Ngan et al found attention and processing deficits in schizophrenia, correlated them with clinically observable psychomotor poverty, and postulated that the negative or deficit symptoms may be clinical manifestations of impaired cognitive processing. Kwon et al found reduced ability to maintain synchronous activity of neuronal firing at higher frequencies—i.e., at 40HZ. Both studies indicate an immaturity of the system consistent with a shift to earlier developmental structures and levels of function.

Gendersen, using electrooculography, found an increased rate of inappropriate saccades in the eye tracking pattern in schizophrenia as opposed to affective or schizoaffective disorders. The baby learns to follow with its eyes at some point in its development but not initially. Thus once more the finding is consistent with a return to a level-of-function/region-of-brain prior to development of the particular ability tested. The age of origin of schizoaffective schizophrenia is at the end of the schizophrenia spectrum, and this is followed by psychotic and then nonpsychotic major depressions. Gendersen's findings therefore indicate that the origin of schizoaffective and affective disorders is after the infant/toddler has gained a capability for smooth eye pursuit.

Meagher et al studied outcome measures and found the longer the patients were left untreated the greater were their negative symptoms and cognitive dysfunctions. This is consistent with more disuse atrophy as the patient uses fewer higher functions for longer periods of time. Kenny et al found that while attention and memory deficits are preeminent in adolescents with schizophrenia, the more global and severe deficits in memory, generative naming and visuospatial and executive functions emerge between adolescence and early adulthood. This too is consistent with a more complete progression into the earlier structures that were active at the time of the original trauma, and with a progressive disuse of the more advanced functions/structures as the person ages.

Maierhofer et al found a reduced discrimination learning capacity, particularly in disorganized as opposed to paranoid schizophrenics, which they attributed to probably a difference in temporal lobe function. Disorganized schizophrenia has an earlier origin than paranoid schizophrenia (as determined by cumulative observations, correlating age of trauma and symptoms). Thus one would expect less discrimination and less temporal lobe development in disorganized schizophrenia because the patient shifts to earlier brain and brain function.

Amar et al found cognitive deficits present in schizophrenia and depression, but found that schizophrenics also exhibit a deficit in free recall. This additional deficit supports the finding that schizophrenia has an earlier age of origin, with a shift to earlier developmental brain structures and more immature levels of function.

Shelley et al found auditory working memory deficits in schizophrenia that were caused by abnormal encoding, and Leiderman et al found accuracy of object working memory, after a five second delay, significantly reduced in schizophrenia over normals—which also was attributed to encoding. Once more the deficits can be attributed to a shift to earlier developmental levels of function and of inputting information.

Ventura et al found neurocognitive deficits in schizophrenia and depression to be the same, but found verbal memory and problem solving impaired in schizophrenia and not in mood disorders. Schizophrenia, for the most part, has its origin prior to the massive development of the language centers, whereas nonpsychotic major depression has its origin later. Thus the impairment in verbal memory should be expected when the patient shifts to the areas of the brain that were active prior to its development.

Jon et al studying QEEG during memory processing found that the frontal and temporal lobes and the thalamus were not appropriately activated in the schizophrenic during memory tasks. This too is consistent with a return to earlier developmental functions and structures and a relative deactivation of those functions/structures that developed later.

Nestor et al, studying MRI and neuropsychological measures, found a positive relation between temporal lobe volume versus verbal learning and categorization, and found a positive relation between frontal lobe volume and performance on attention and working memory tasks. In schizophrenia, the volumes and functions of both are reduced—which is precisely what one would expect when a schizophrenic patient shifts to the structures/functions that were active prior to the development of language centers in the left posterior superior temporal gyrus and prior to the massive development of the frontal lobes.

MacQueen et al found patients with acute psychosis have impairment in selective attention. More acute illness equates with a greater shift of activity away from the frontal lobes.

Levitt et al conducted important MRI studies that revealed an *increase in brain stem absolute volume* among schizophrenics as opposed to normals—which supports the concept of a shift of activity to the phylogenetically earlier brain structures, resulting in an increase in volume and an increase in neurotransmitters produced there. They also found an increase in cerebellum white matter, an increase in vermian gray and especially white matter, and an increase in vermian anterior lobule volume. Considering the fact that the schizophrenic was traumatized at about the time he was learning to walk, when the growth and development of the cerebellum was at its peak, the increase in activity there—along with the increase in volume (as occurs in any structure that is exercised)—gives further support to the concept of a shift of activity to the function/structure that was developing at the time/age of the original trauma.

Downhill et al (1997a) found an increase in corpus callosum size which correlated with an increase in symptoms of schizophrenia, and found that a smaller corpus callosum was associated with a greater left-right asymmetry in the cingulate, suggesting an increase in interhemispheric communication between left and right cingulate which was proportionate to an increase in symptoms of schizophrenia. The findings might indicate a compensatory mechanism caused by the reduced size [activity] (Fodor) in the schizophrenic's right cingulate—which would require greater utilization of the left cingulate to compensate for inactivity on the right, and thereby increase the size of the corpus callosum. This compensatory mechanism is one the author suggested to Richard Petty for his finding of an increase in size of the right posterior superior temporal gyrus in the schizophrenic (personal communication, 1996). If a person loses the use of one arm, for example, the other becomes more developed.

Downhill et al (1997b) identified a decreased temporal lobe volume in both schizotypal personality disorder and in schizophrenia. Both these disorders have origins prior to the massive development of the speech centers in the left posterior superior temporal gyrus, and a return to brain structures that were active prior to that massive development would account for the disuse atrophy.

Byne et al found that thalamic volume loss varied from 5% to 33% depending on subdivision of the thalamus. Crosson determined that the dominant thalamus is involved in verbal working memory, and that the deficit lies in the interface between semantic and lexical systems. Both logically would result from a shift to brain structures that were active prior to the massive development of the language centers, with a disuse atrophy of later developmental structures.

Jeste et al found that late onset schizophrenia had less impairment in learning, larger thalamic volume and smaller volume of lenticular nucleus as compared to early onset. The less severe impairment in learning correlates with less disuse atrophy in the dominant thalamus which is involved in verbal working memory. Other variables may apply to late onset schizophrenia, and the findings should be studied in light of the overall pattern that is emerging—i.e., 1) activation of specific earlier developmental structures and functions, depending on time/age of original trauma, 2) disuse atrophy of later developmental structures/functions and the pathways they use, 3) the development of neuronal pathways interconnecting the structures that are active, and 4) changes that are proportionate to intensity and duration of illness, which may include structural changes based on growth of unconscious core nuclei of conscious prior to the initial awakening of the delayed Posttraumatic Stress Disorder mechanism.

Buchsbaum et al (1997a) found significantly lower metabolic rates in the mediodorsal nucleus of the left thalamus, which is a major cortical relay from the limbic system and has connections to the prefrontal cortex. This is consistent with disuse of the prefrontal cortex, an area of brain which develops largely after the age of origin of schizophrenia.

Shihabuddin et al found a significant difference in metabolic rate between Kraepelinian and non-Kraepelinian schizophrenia. Disorders that are allowed to progress simply do so. Many of the back ward Schizophrenic patients of yesteryear no longer are seen in such great numbers simply because the natural progression of the illness has been interrupted.

Ghanem et al, correlating SPECT and WCST, found Schizophrenics with more negative symptoms had a greater decrease in rCBF in the right frontal, temporal and right and left parietal lobes, while a decrease in left frontal rCBF occurred equally with positive or negative symptoms. Cumulative observations correlating age of origin with symptoms reveal a progressive and substantial reduction in affect among those traumatized prior to 18 months. Thus a patient with more negative symptoms would have an origin prior to those with more positive symptoms, and would use earlier developmental brain structures. Negative symptomotology also may reflect further progression into the illness.

Gupta et al, using MRI coregistered with PET, found a positive correlation between ventricular volume and duration of the illness, and a significant negative correlation between ventricular volume and metabolic rate—in the angular gyrus and the primary visual cortex. These changes are consistent with disuse, as would occur in any other part of the body.

Buchsbaum et al (1997b), utilizing a new visualization technique for analyzing white matter tracts, demonstrated evidence of diminished communication in frontostriatal pathways in schizophrenia. Since there is relatively less activity in the frontal cortex, it should be expected that interconnecting pathways would be atrophied.

Quinn et al, studying histopathology of glial archectecture of human cortex, found a disruption of caudate astrocyte function and hypothesized this could have neurocognitive sequellae in schizophrenia. While this is true, the high correlation with infant trauma indicates that the disruption of caudate astrocyte function more likely is caused by the schizophrenic process, and in accordance with the mechanisms described.

Kang et al, found an alteration in monoamine metabolism, especially in female schizophrenics with symptoms of depression and anxiety, and Gerdsen et al found a hemispheric asymmetry of benzodiazepine receptor binding sites in schizophrenia, using SPECT. While these changes are a part of a chain of reactions which cause other reactions to occur, the high correlation between infant traumas and the later development of the disorder leads one to suspect that it is the trauma that sets the process in motion.

Murray, in the Adolph Meyer Award Lecture, summarizes current thinking, attributing early onset schizophrenia to neurodevelopmental impairment. Neurostructural changes are present, but it is not yet determined what portion may be precursor versus what portion is the result of the disease process. The high correlation between schizophrenia and infant traumas indicate most brain changes more likely are the result of the disease process and not the cause. Age of onset is viewed by the present author more as a function of when the precipitating trauma occurred, but it is recognized that *the more vulnerable the individual the sooner he encounters a trauma that can awaken the earlier traumatic gestalt*. Murray attributes familial cases to a genetic defect in control of development of normal cortical asymmetry. This transposition is commonplace, but it may be in error. Familial is not genetic until proven to be so. Murray cites prenatal and perinatal factors, such as viral infections and hypoxia, postulating that the dysplastic neural network may be responsible for delayed milestones in preschizophrenic children, and acknowledging that it is not known whether the abnormal factors are the cause of the process or whether they are risk factors for it. Indeed the pre and perinatal factors might alter structure but can also serve as the antecedent traumas that cause the infant traumas to be experienced as more severe. Both would represent risk factors.

DATA FROM FEBRUARY 1998 NINTH BIENNIAL WINTER WORKSHOP ON SCHIZOPHRENIA IN DAVOS, SWITZERLAND:

Devoted exclusively to schizophrenia, the conference hosted approximately 75 lectures and 500 poster presentations describing the latest research findings. It would be redundant to review each one, but to the author, none of the biological findings appeared incongruous with a shift of brain activity to earlier developmental structures.

To mention but a few, the schizophrenic loses normal asymmetry (Purdon, Zaidel, Crow) [because there is a shift of brain activity to an age prior to the development of specialization]. Brain atrophy relates to smaller cells, not fewer (Garey) [indicating disuse atrophy, not cell death]. There is an increase in size of lamina II pyramidal cells in the entorhinal cortex

(Longson) [because of increased activity in this earlier developmental layer].

SUMMARY:

The view of the present author is that genetic factors represent predisposition to schizophrenia and other disorders, and eventually the precise level of contribution will be determined.

Pre and perinatal factors along with obstetric and birth traumas represent antecedent traumas, setting the stage for subsequent traumas to be more severe, and they also can impact directly on brain development. Infant separation traumas—because they represented death to the mammalian species for 150 million years—are much more significant than previously suspected, and set the stage for the later development of delayed Posttraumatic Stress Disorders.

In delayed PTSD, a second trauma, similar to the first, partially awakens the entire earlier gestalt, setting the process in motion. The flashback is to the earlier mind/brain/reality/feelings/behavior/chemistry/physiology and neuroanatomical sites that were active at the time/age of the original trauma, and from this reactivation of earlier sites there is a release of neurotransmitters produced by those sites or through the reactivation of those sites; there is the development of aberrant neuronal pathways which interconnect the new areas of activity; and there is disuse atrophy of the later developmental structures and their interconnecting pathways—as would occur in any other part of the body not used.

Any stressor can cause intensification of the original trauma or of the subsequent trauma that reactivates the earlier gestalt. This can include anything in the environment that causes stress. Viral factors might fit into this category or might be noncausally related.

The important research findings presented in San Diego (1997) and in Davos (1998) are more meaningful when viewed under one roof and in relation to one another. There has been an explosion of knowledge in recent decades, with each particle moving farther from the core. Without a unified working model, professionals and lay persons alike are left with isolated concepts that schizophrenia is a chemical imbalance, or a genetic disorder, or a brain disease, or a biopsychosocial disorder, or many diseases with many causes. Each finding instead must be integrated within the framework of one unified construct in order to bring understanding to a new level. Genetics can be viewed as predisposition, with biochemical, structural and psychosocial change viewed primarily as the result of a single disease process. The concept of delayed Posttraumatic Stress Disorders from infancy, with a partial shift of activity to earlier mind/brain/reality/feelings/behavior/chemistry/physiology and neuroanatomic sites, and the resultant interaction of that earlier gestalt with adult brain functions/structures, may be the best working model we have at the present time for integrating and understanding all the complexities of the disease process. O. Spurgeon English, in his Foreword to McKenzie and Wright (1996), referred to this model as "the new unification theory of mental illness."

It is hoped that this work, in addition to bringing fourth new understanding to serious mental/emotional disorders, will help unify the field and bring the many disciplines together. The process of unification already is taking place slowly, one study at a time, as newer studies coregister PET with MRI and bring in neuropsychological testing, for example, but the field can advance exponentially, with the pieces of the puzzle rapidly falling into place, if there is a structural framework that enables each researcher to maintain a larger view and understand his or her contribution in relation to the entire disease process. The new unification theory, backed by research studies and references in the literature, is the most inclusive model at the present time, and provides a clear, equal and logical place for each discipline.

BIBLIOGRAPHY

Amar, G., Fossati, P.H., Raoux, No., Allilaire, J.F. (1997) Memory Processes & Executive Functions in Depression and Schizophrenia. APA Meeting, May, 1997, San Diego.

Bettelheim, B. (1967). *The Empty Fortress*: Infantile Autism and the Birth of Self. Collier MacMillan Ltd. London. 484 pps. The autistic anlage, p. 39-47; The right side of time, p. l 47-57; Extreme situations, p. 63-68; In lieu of evidence, p. 351-366; Feral or autistic, p. 367-372.

Bettelheim, B. (1969). *The Children of the Dream: Infancy and Early Childhood*. Collier MacMillan Ltd. London. 363 pps. Desertion, p. 92; The impermanent adult, p. 100; Autonomy, shame, doubt, p. 307.

Borus, J.F. (1973). Reentry: I. Adjustment issues facing the Vietnam returnee. *Arch. Gen. Psychiatry* 28: 501-506.

Breier, A.F. (1994). Dopamine, Stress & Schizophrenia. APA Meeting, May, 1994, Philadelphia.

Buchsbaum, M.S., Hazlett, E.A., Haznadar, M.M., Geneve, C., Shihabuddin, L.S. (1997a). Three Dimensional Analysis of Thalamic Metabolic Rate in Schizophrenia. APA Meeting, May, 1997, San Diego.

Buchsbaum, M.S., Tang, C.Y., Hazlett, E.A., Lu, D., Spiegel-Cohen, M.S., Atlas, S.W. (1997b). Diffusion Tensor Analysis of White Matter pathways in Schizophrenia. APA Meeting, May, 1997, San Diego.

Byne, W., Jones, L., Kemether, E., Haroutunian, V., Davis, K.L. (1997). Toward Localization of Thalamic Pathology in Schizophrenia. APA Meeting, May, 1997, San Diego.

Crosson, B. (1997). The Thalamic in Language on Neurocognition. APA Meeting, May, 1997, San Diego.

Crow, T.J. (1990). Brain Structure in Psychosis and the Descent of Man. APA meeting, May 1990, New York.

Crow, T.J. (1998). A Bi-hemispheric Theory of the origin of Schneiderian Nuclear Symptoms. Ninth Biennial Winter Workshop on Schizophrenia. February, 1998. Davos.

Doman, G. (1974). *What to do About Your Brain Injured Child.* 1982 edition. The Better Baby Press, with Doubleday & Co., 291 pps.

Doman, G. (1984). *How to Give Your Baby Encyclopedia Knowledge.* The Better Baby Press, Philadelphia. 302 pps.

Downhill, J.E., Buchsbaum, M.S., Haznadar, M., Wei, T.C., Spiegel-Cohen, J. (1997a). Relationship Between Corpus Callosum Size, Cingulate Gyrus Metabolic Rate and Symptoms of Schizophrenia. APA Meeting, May, 1997, San Diego.

Downhill, J.E., Buchsbaum, M.S., Hazlett, E.A., Barth, S., Lees-Roitman, S., Nunn, M., Seiver, L.J. (1997b). Temporal Lobe Volume in Schizotypical Personality Disorder and Schizophrenia. APA Meeting, May, 1997, San Diego.

Eth, S., and Pynoos, R. (1985). Post-traumatic Stress Disorder in Children, *American Psychiatric Press*, Washington, D.C.

Fodor, P.A., Sheeder, J., Rohas, D.C., Teale, P.D., Simon, J., Reite, M.L. (1997). Volumetric Comparisons of the Cingulate Gyrus in Patients with Schizophrenia and Controls. APA Meeting, May, 1997, San Diego.

Freud, A. (1953). Some remarks on infant observation. Psychoanalytic Study of the Child. Vol. VIII. *International Universities Press*, New York, pp. 9-19.

Freud, S. (1926). *The Problem of Anxiety*, Norton, New York.

Gampel, Y. (1988). Facing war, murder, torture and death in latency. *Psychoana. Rev.* 75.

Gampel, Y. (1989). I was a Holocaust Child. In Wilson, A. (ed.), The Holocaust Survivor and the Family, In press.

Garey, L.J., Radewicz, K., Reynolds, R. (1998). Increase in Microglia in Frontal and Temporal Cortex of Schizophrenics. Ninth Biennial Winter Workshop on Schiozphrenia. February, 1998. Davos.

Gerdsen, I. (1997a). Difference of Eye Tracking Pattern in Schizophrenia, Affective and Schizoaffective Disorders: A Lab Investigation Using Electrooculography. APA Meeting, May, 1997, San Diego.

Gerdsen, I., Pinkert, J., Oehme, L., Ripke, B., Zoephal, K., Newmann, V. (1997b). Hemispheric Asymmetry of Benzodiazepine Receptor Binding Sites in Schizophrenia: A Study with I-Lomazenil SPECT. APA Meeting, May, 1997, San Diego.

Ghanem, M.H., Kamel, M., Sadek, A., El-Banauby, M., Kwalil, S. (1997). SPECT in Schizophrenics with Positive Versus Negative Symptoms. APA Meeting, May, 1997, San Diego.

Gupta, A.K., Buchsbaum, M.S., Hazlett, E.A. (1997). Left Ventricular Size Increases with Age and is Associated with Reduced Parietal and Occipital Cortical Metabolic Rate in Schizophrenia. APA Meeting, May, 1997, San Diego.

Harlow, H.F., and Woolsey, C.N. (1958). Biological and Biochemical Bases of Behavior. *Halstead Press*, pps. 355-357, 425-467.

Harlow, H.F. (1979). *The Human Model: Primate Perspectives*. Halstead Press.

Hazlett, E.A., Buchsbaum, M.S., Haznadar, M.M., Biren, M., Schnur, D.B. (1997). Frontal Lobe and Startle Eye-Blink Deficits in Schizophrenia. APA Meeting, May, 1997, San Diego.

Hyman, I.A., Zeikoff, W., and Clarke, J. (1988). Psychological and physical abuse in the schools: A paradigm for understanding post-traumatic stress disorder in children and youth. *Journal of Traumatic Stress*, Vol. 1, No. 2, p. 243.

Janet, P. (1886). Les actes inconscients et la memoire pendant le somnambulisme. *Rev. Philos.* 25(I): 238-279.

Janet, P. (1919). *Les medications psychologiques* (3 volumes), Alcan, Paris.

Jeste, D.V., Symonds, L.L., Jernigan, T.L., Stout, J., Braff, D.L., Heaton, R.K. (1997). Thalamus and Late-Life Schizophrenia. APA Meeting, May, 1997, San Diego.

Jon, D-I., Lee, S.H., Lee, H-S., Min, S.K. (1997). QEEG During Memory Tasks in Schizophrenia. APA Meeting, May, 1997, San Diego.

Kang, D-Y., Poole, J., Vinogradov, S., Willis-Shore, J., Corwin, F., Lieberman, M., Marco, E. (1997). Relationships Among Psychopathology, Gender and Monamine Metabolism in Chronic Schizophrenia. APA Meeting, May, 1997, San Diego.

Kardiner, A. (1941). *The Traumatic Neuroses of War*. Psychosomatic Medicine Monograph II-III, National Research Council, Washington, D.C.

Kenny, J.T., Friedman, L., Findling, R.L., Swales, T.P., Strauss, M.E., Schultz, S.C. (1997). Cognitive Impairment in Adolescent Schizophrenia. APA Meeting, May, 1997, San Diego.

Kestenberg, J.S. (1987). Imagining and remembering. Unpublished paper, Sands Point, New York.

Kestenberg, J.S., and Brenner, I. (1986). Children who survived the holocaust. *Int. J. Psychanal.* 67:309-316.

Kilpatrick, D.G., Veronen, L.J.l, and Best, C.L. (1985). Factors predicting psychological distress among rape victims. In Figley, C.R. (ed.), *Trauma and Its Wake*, Brunner/Mazel, New York, pp. 113-141.

Kraemer, G.W., Ebert, M.H., Lake, C.R., and McKinney, G.W. (1984). Hypersensitivity to d-amphetamine several years after early social deprivation in rhesus monkeys, *Psychopharmacology* 82: 266-271.

Krystal, J.H., Larvelle, M., Abi-Darghaur, A., Seibyl, J.P., Karpour, L.P., Charney, D.S. (1994). Serotonin and Schizophrenia. APA Meeting, May, 1994, Philadelphia.

Kwon, J.S., O'Donnell, B.F., McCarley, B.W., Gurrera, R.J., Greene, R.W., Hirayasu, Y. (1997). Reduced Response of Auditory Steady State 40 HZ in Schizophrenia. APA Meeting, May, 1997, San Diego.

Leiderman, E.A., Strejilevich, S.A., de Lajonquiere, C.A. (1997). Working Memory Dysfunction in Schizophrenics. APA Meeting, May, 1997, San Diego.

Levitt, J.J., Donnino, R.M., Shenton, M.E., Kikinis, R., Jolesz, F.A., McCurley, R.W. (1997). The Cerebellum, Vermis and Brainstem in Schizophrenia: An MRI Study. APA Meeting, May, 1997, San Diego.

Longson, D., Longson, C.M., Deakin, J.F.W., Benes, F.M. (1998). Specific Increase in Size of Lamina II Pyrimedal Cells in the Entorhinal Cortex in Schizophrenia. Ninth Biennial Winter Workshop on Schizophrenia. February, 1998. Davos.

MacLean, P.D. (1973). *A Triune Concept of the Brain and Behavior.* The Clarence M. Hicks Memorial Lectures 1969 for Ontario Mental Health Foundation, University of Toronto Press, 165 pps.

MacLean, P.D. (1985). Brain evolution relating to family, play and the separation call. *Arch. Gen. Psychiat.* 42: 505-417.

MacQueen, G., Rosebush, P.E., Tipper, S. (1997). Deficits in Visual Selective Attention in Neuroleptic Naïve Psychotic Patients Versus Nonpsychiatric Controls. APA Meeting, May, 1997, San Diego.

Mahler, M.S. (1979). *The Selected Papers of Margaret S. Mahler, M.D.* (2 vols.). V. Aronson Publisher, New York, 242 pps.

Maierhofer, D., Dantendorfer, K., Hofer, E., Serim, M., Windhaber, J., Katschnigs, H. (1997). Condition Discrimination Learning in Schizophrenia. APA Meeting, May, 1997, San Diego.

Malhorta, A.K., Su, T.P., Kammerer, W., Pickar, D., Breier, A.F. (1994) Glutamatergic Hypothesis of Schizophrenia. APA Meetings, May 1994, Philadelphia.

McKenzie, C. (1981). *Schizophrenia and the McKenzie Method.* Audio Tape Cassettes. American Health Association. Box 345, Bala Cynwyd, PA.

McKenzie, C. (1984). *The Anatomy & Psychodynamics of Psychosis.* Lecture, International Congress in Madrid. Monograph, American Health Association, Box 345, Bala Cynwyd, PA.

McKenzie, C. (1986). Having Schizophrenia is Unnecessary. Lecture Series at the Philadelphia County Medical Society.

McKenzie, C., Wright, L. (1996). Delayed Posttraumatic Stress Disorders from Infancy: The Two Trauma Mechanism. Harwood Academic Press. Distributed by U. of Toronto Press. 225 pgs.

Meagher, D.J., Waddington, J.L., Millaney, J., Quissen, J.J., Murphy, P. (1997). Outcome Measures in Initially Untreated Psychosis. APA Meeting, May, 1997, San Diego.

Nemeroff, C.B. (1993). The Psychoneuroendocrinology of Depression: Hypothalamic-Pituitary-Adrenal Axis Dysregulation. Strecker Monograph Series XXX, November, 1993, Institute of the Pennsylvania Hospital, Philadelphia.

Nemeroff, C.B. (1994). Neuropeptides and schizophrenia. APA Meeting, May, 1994, Philadelphia.

Nestor, P.G., Barnard, J., O'Donnell, B.F., Shenton, M.E., Kikinis, R. Joelsz, F.A. (1997). MRI and Neuropsychological Measures in Schizophrenia: Partial Least Squares Analysis. APA Meeting, May, 1997, San Diego.

Ngan, E.T.C., Liddle, P.F. (1997). Attention and Information Processing Deficits in Schizophrenia: Correlate with Clinical Syndromes. APA Meeting, May, 1997, San Diego.

Pascwani, A., Bartlett, E., Duncan, E., Madonic, S.H., Chappell, P.B., Rajan, R. (1997). Gating in Schizophrenia: A Trait-Related Deficit. APA Meeting, May, 1997, San Diego.

Pearce, J.C. (1977). *Magical Child*. E.P. Dutton, New York.

Pearce, J.C. (1985). *Magical Child Matures*. E.P. Dutton, New York, 235 pps.

Purdon, S.E., Pasmeny, G., Doerkson, S., & Waldie, B. (1998). Lateralized Olfactory Acuity Deficits and Olfactory Misidentification in Schizophrenia. Ninth Biennial Winter Workshop on Schizophrenia. February, 1998. Davos.

Pynoos, R., and Eth, S. (1985). Developmental perspectives on psychic trauma. In Figley, C.R. (ed.), *Trauma and Its Wake*, Brunner/Mazel, New York, pp. 36-52.

Quinn, B., Byne, W.M., Conklin, L.S., Davis, K.L. (1997). Glial Architecture of Human Cortex: Implications for Neurocognition in Schizophrenia. APA Meeting, May, 1997, San Diego.

Raifman, L.J. (1983). Problems of diagnosis and legal causation in courtroom use of post-traumatic stress disorder. *Behav. Sci. Law* 1(3): 115-130.

Samuel, T. (1990). Vietnam's delayed hit. *Philadelphia Inquirer*, May 28, 1990, p. E-1.

Shelley, A-M., Javitt, D.C., Vaughn, H.G. (1997). Working Memory Dysfunction in Schizophrenia. APA Meeting, May, 1997, San Diego.

Shihabuddin, L.S., Buchsbaum, M.S., Hazlett, E.A., Schroeder, J., Haznadar, M.M., Davis, K.L. (1997). Metabolic Rate in Kraepelinian Versus Non-Kraepelinian Schizophrenia. APA Meeting, May, 1997, San Diego.

Spitz, R. (1945). Hospitalism: An inquiry into the genesis of psychiatric conditions in early childhood. *Psychoanalytic Study Child* I: 53-74.

Spitz, R.A., Cobliner, W.G. (1975). Emotional deficiency diseases of the infant. The First Year of Life. *International Universities Press*, pps. 267-300.

van der Kolk, B.A. (1988). The trauma spectrum: The interaction of biological and social events in the genesis of the trauma response. *Journal of Traumatic Stress*, Vol. 1, No. 3, p.l 277-279.

van der Kolk, B.A., and Ducey, C.P. (1984). Clinical implications of the Rorschach in post-traumatic stress disorder. In van der Kolk, B.A. (ed.), Post-Traumatic Stress Disorder: Psychological and Biological Sequelae, *American Psychiatric Press*, Washington.

van der Kolk, B.A., and Ducey, C.P. (1989). The psychological processing of traumatic experience. Rorschach patterns in PTSD. *Journal of Traumatic Stress*, Vol. 2, No. 3, p. 265-267.

van der Ploeg, H.M., and Kleijn, W.C. (1989). Being held hostage in the Netherlands: A study of long-term aftereffects. *Journal of Traumatic Stress*, Vol. 2, No. 2, p. 154, 166.

van Kammen, D.P., Gurklis, J.A., Peters, J.L., Kelly, P.A., Yao, J.K. (1994). A Role of Norepinephrins in Schizophrenia. APA Meeting, May, 1994, Philadelphia.

Ventura, D., McMillis, W., Guze, B.H., Humphrey, L., Gitlin, M.J. (1997). Neuropsychology of Mood Disorder and Schizophrenia Disorder. APA Meeting, May, 1997, San Diego.

Williams, J.S., and Siegel, J.P. (1989). Marital disruption and physical illness: The impact of divorce and spouse death on illness. *Journal of Traumatic Stress*, Vol. 2, No. 4, p. 555.

Willis-Shore, J., Vinogradov, S., Poole, J., Ober, B.A., Shenaut, G. (1997). Slower Reaction Time in Schizophrenia: Relationship to Clinical Symptoms and Cerebral Dysfunction. APA Meeting, May, 1997, San Diego.

Zaidel, D.W.(1998). Evidence for Hemispheric Symmetry in Schizophrenia from Computer Measurements in Postmortem Tissues of Left and Right Hippocampus. Ninth Biennial Winter Workshop on Schizophrenia. February, 1998. Davos.

Zelikoff, W. (1986). Evidence for a new diagnostic construct: Educator-induced post traumatic stress disorder. Unpublished manuscript, Temple University, Philadelphia.

Index

A

AA (Alcoholics Anonymous), 151
"abscess" of the mind, 8, 24, 26, 30-35, 37-39, 41
ADD (attention deficit disorder), 135
ADHD (attention deficit hyperactivity disorder), 3, 116-17, 134-35
adoption, 126-27, 256
adoption agencies, 127, 256
AEC (Atomic Energy Commission), 78-79
alcohol, 115, 137, 160, 215
  dependence, 3, 116, 136, 145
alcoholism, 45, 107, 137, 156, 269-70
Ali, Abdullah Yusuf, 82
allergic reactions, 232-33
alpha brain wave frequency, 60, 195-96
Amar, G., 274
American Journal of Psychiatry, 49, 193
American Psychiatric Association, 50, 90
Amundsen, Roald, 58
"Anatomy and Psychodynamics of Psychosis, The" (McKenzie), 48, 266

angels, 244
anger, 69, 184, 205, 208-10. *See also* depression
anhedonia, 215
anorexia, 138-39, 168
anoxia, 98
antecedent traumas, 47, 112, 278-79
Anthony, Casey, 84
anxiety, 188, 197, 214-15, 250
  castration, 251
  depression and, 214-15, 217
  in PTSD, 4, 9, 144-45
apathy, 184, 187, 217-19. *See also* need
arthritis, 230
asthma, 133
Atomic Energy Commission, 78-79
atrophy, 267
  brain, 47, 52, 102-3, 267, 278
  disuse, 103, 105, 154, 268, 272-73, 276, 279
  muscle, 231
attachment, 206-7
attention deficit disorder, 135
attention deficit hyperactivity disorder, iv, 3, 116-17, 134-35
aura, 66-67, 205, 207-8

autism, 116-19, 256, 269
automatic pilot, 7, 20, 45, 96. *See also*
    survival mechanism
avoidance phenomena, 21, 23
awareness, 67, 74, 145, 200-201, 224,
    233
  conscious, 7-8, 24
  meditation and, 246
  prior to birth, 255

B

babies, 9, 97, 124
  adopted, 127-28
  feeding, 257
  Moro reflex in, 100
  mothers and, 114, 127
  separated from mother, 18, 20, 52,
    96, 111, 121, 128
  traumas to, 22
Baxter, Cleve, 260
Beautiful Mind, A, 20, 162
Bedrij, Orest, 78-79
  *Celebrate Your Divinity: The
    Nature of God and the Theory of
    Everything*, 80
  *'I': The Foundation and
    Mathematization of Physics*, 80
behavior, 10
  change in, 146
  infant, 10, 48, 265
  strange, 9, 23, 45, 149
  violent, 130
Bettelheim, Bruno, xiv, 119, 268
Bhagavad Gita, 219
biofeedback, 201, 223
biological change, 47, 50, 115, 118,
    263-65, 267
bipolar disorder, 171, 194

bipolar hypomania, 133
birth, 98-101, 266
  trauma, 47, 98, 112
birth of a sibling, 120
  delayed PTSD and, 114, 265
  schizophrenia and, 103, 149,
    177-78
  time within, 110
body movements, 16, 48, 97
borderline personality disorders,
    126-27, 135, 256
brain
  activity, 54, 134, 257
  atrophy, 47, 102-3, 267, 278
  damage, 98
Brown, G. W., 160
Buchsbaum, M. S., 276-77
Burlingham, Dorothy, 89
Byne, W., 276

C

Cancro, Robert, 49, 107
cannibalism, 139
castration anxiety, 251
catatonic schizophrenia, 102, 112,
    123, 181
Cayce, Edgar, 239
*Celebrate Your Divinity: The Nature of
    God and the Theory of Everything*
    (Bedrij), 80
cerebellum, 101, 275
Chidananda, Swami, 80-81, 226
childhood schizophrenia, vii, 15, 72,
    119, 269
child protection agencies, 127-28
Christians, 82, 152, 200, 207, 216,
    226, 257
chronic fatigue syndrome, 236

circumcision, 48, 117, 256
clinical significance, 49. *See also* statistical significance
cognitive impairment, 102
combat reality, 5, 24, 104, 265
combat veteran
  maladaptive mode of the, 21
  PTSD and the, 26, 96, 103, 153
  shift to infant reality of the, 46, 264
  shift to war experience of the, 5, 97, 102, 269
conscious awareness, 7-8, 24
consciousness, 89, 91, 256
  core nucleus of, 35, 37, 270
  levels of, 60, 191, 196, 198, 202, 222
  meditation and, 195
corpus callosum, 101, 275
Crosson, B., 276
Crow, Timothy, 110, 268

D

Dalai Lama, 238
Daniel (Jewish prophet), 245, 248
David (king of Israel), 87
Davidson, Gerald E., 126
DeCani, John, vii, 104, 271
defense mechanisms, 6
Delayed Posttraumatic Stress Disorders from Infancy (McKenzie and Wright), xv, 12, 20, 162, 263-64, 280
depression, 133, 149, 152-53, 184, 188, 205, 214
  anxiety and, 215
  avoiding, 100
  cause of, 266
  grief-related, 189
  incidence of, 113
  major, xiii, 146, 188, 215, 263, 266, 270-71, 273-74
  nonpsychotic, 26, 53, 100, 105, 133-34, 150
  prevention of, 52
  psychotic, 26, 53
  suicidal, 133, 159-60, 189
  treatment of, 183-85, 217
  See also anger
desire, 67, 183-84, 205, 209-11, 214. *See also* need
developmental brain reflexes, age of origin of, 100
Diagnostic and Statistical Manual, 93
Diamond, John, 84-85
Diamond, Susan, 84
disorganized schizophrenia, 128, 273-74
disuse atrophy, 103, 105, 267, 272, 276
Doman, G., 266
dopamine, 46, 52, 102-3, 267
Downhill, J. E., 275
dream, 31, 68, 190, 223, 228
Dr. Laura. *See* Schlessinger, Laura
drug addiction, 137, 237
drugs, 115, 125, 155, 176, 189
Ducey, C. P., 269
dyslexia, 136, 149

E

eating disorders, 3, 49, 138
EE (expressed emotion) factor, 160-61, 167, 184
Ego and the Id, The (Freud), 220
ego needs, 187, 191, 216, 248, 259
Einstein, Albert, xvii, 58, 79, 108

emotional separation trauma, 20, 46, 162
emotional transformation therapy, 191
emotions, 130
energy, 207, 217-20
  desire and, 67
  emotional, 8, 34
  negative, 209-10, 215
  positive, 208, 215
English, O. Spurgeon, 49, 71, 88, 147, 206, 216, 280
enlightenment, iv, viii, 84, 168, 203, 222, 233, 249
ETT (emotional transformation therapy), 191
exercise, 185, 200-201, 204
existence, 79
existential analysis. See logotherapy
exorcism, 90
Exorcist, The, 90
Ezekiel (Hebrew prophet), 158

F

failure-to-thrive syndrome, 145
fear, 91, 97-98, 215, 221, 225
feeding, 257-58
fetus, 109
Figley, Charles, 49
flashback, 29, 32, 53, 104
  hallucinatory, 5
  initial, 19, 104
  separation and, 146, 263
forgiveness, 69, 167, 208, 215-17
Frankl, Viktor, 187
Freud, Anna, xiv, 89, 268
Freud, Sigmund, xvii, 59, 76, 220, 268
  dreams and, 245

Ego and the Id, The, 220
  introspection of, 59
  on intuition, 76
  observations of, 89
  on war neuroses, 112
Friedman, Milton, 238-39

G

Gabrielli violin, 85. See also Peresson violin
Gallagher, Fr. Eugene, 90
gall bladder, 227
Gandhi, Mahatma, 108
genetic research, 13, 129
genetic weakness, 106, 108
Ghanem, M. H., 277
God, 67, 79, 125, 199, 212, 225, 257
Great Spirit, 81. See also Holy Spirit
Green, Elmer, 201, 223, 232
  Ozawkie Book of the Dead, The, 223
guiding power, 76, 92
gun, 21, 130, 132, 153, 264
gunas, 219
  rajas, 219
  sattva, 219
  tamas, 219
Gupta, A. K., 277

H

hallucinatory flashback, 5
happiness, 205-6, 211-12, 258
hate, 150, 210
Hearne, Ronald, 70
hebephrenic schizophrenia, 128
Heidnik, Gary, 139, 148
hippocampus, 103, 105
Hitler, Adolf, 130

Holy Spirit, 81, 200. *See also* Great Spirit
Hussein, Saddam, 130, 239
hypoglycemia, 134-35

I

IBM, 78-79
idiot savants, 138
idol worship, 80
ileocecal junction, 229-30
inescapable shock, 6-7
infancy, 18, 21, 125
   shift to, 96, 217
   trauma during, 104-5, 122, 266
infant separation
   social factors leading to, 131
   trauma, 263, 268, 279
infant traumas, 16, 19, 105, 115, 122
Influenza Virus, 109-10
initial flashback, 19, 104
intestinal obstruction, 229-30
intestinal tract, 229-30
Isaiah (Hebrew prophet), 51, 87, 125

J

Janet, Pierre, 35
Jeremiah (Hebrew prophet), 158, 211
Jeste, D. V., 276
John Paul II (pope), 81
Jon, D-I, 274
Journal of Traumatic Stress, 49

K

Kang, D-Y, 277
Kardiner, A., 266
Kekulé, Friedrich August, xvii
Kenny, J. T., 273
Kissinger, Henry, 239
Kraemer, G. W., 269
Kraepelinian schizophrenia, 276
Kripalvananda, Swami, 83
Kuhlman, Kathryn, 82

L

language
   centers, 101-2, 265, 272, 274, 276
   development, 101-2, 109, 268
Leiderman, E. A., 274
Levitt, J. J., 275
Lewin, Bertram, 139
light therapy, 184, 188
light treatment, 185
Littleton High School, 130
liver failure, 137-38
logotherapy, 187
lotus position, 67, 71, 196
love energy
   how to increase, 212
   in therapy, 214
lux, 184-85

M

MacLean, Paul, xiv, 18, 48, 266, 268
MacQueen, G., 275
magnesium, 135
Mahler, Margaret, vii, xiv, 15, 48, 72, 119, 269
Maierhofer, D., 273
major depressive episode, 22, 45, 154, 189
malnutrition, 109
manic-type bipolar disorder, 133
Maya trap, 206

McKenzie, Christina (younger daughter of CM and DM), viii, 60, 62, 225
McKenzie, Clancy (CM), xv, 12, 20, 162, 263-64, 280
  Delayed Posttraumatic Stress Disorders from Infancy, xv, 12, 20, 162, 263-64, 280
  exploring the unknown, 58
  formal education of, 59
  hearing a powerful, authoritative voice during sleep, 62
  meditation of, 228
  three idols of, 58
  witnessing shooting stars, 64-65
  writing about love energy, 66
McKenzie, Dianna (DM), 60, 74
McKenzie, Helen (mother of CM), 57
McKenzie, Hughie (father of CM), 57
McKenzie, Victoria (first daughter of CM and DM), viii, 60-62
Meagher, D. J., 273
Medical Tribune, 166
medications, 125, 138, 192
  effectiveness of, 193
  elimination of, 156
  recovery and, 193
meditation, 60, 186, 195, 213, 246
  deep, 202-3, 223
  exercises, 200
  intuitive voice during, 76
  light level of, 60, 65, 195-97, 199-200, 202
  peace in, 214
Mednick, Sarnoff, vii, xv, 49, 53, 110, 272
Menninger, Karl, 88
mental illness, 3, 249
  cause and mechanism of, 146
  prevention and treatment of, 92, 118
  unification model for, xiv, 103, 115, 263-64, 280
  unification theory of, xiv, 263, 280
mercury, 117, 231
migration, 113, 123
Mike (reverend), 72-74
mineral depletion, 134-35
Monroe, Marilyn, 150
Moro reflex, 100, 265
Mortensen, Preben Bo, 53, 111-12
motherhood, 146, 253-54
mothers, 20, 44, 52, 114, 117, 131, 135, 162, 207, 225, 253
  alcoholic, 136-37
  babies' emotional separation from, 18-20
  love of, 253-54
Mother Teresa, 206
Murray, Robin, 278

N

NAMI (National Alliance for Mental Illness), 51
Nash, John, vii, 20, 162
National Alliance for Mental Illness, 51
natural childbirth education, 255-56
Nebuchadnezzar, King, 248
need, 183-84, 187, 205, 210, 214. *See also* desire
negative energy, 209-10, 215-16
negative programming, 247
Nemeroff, C. B., 266-67
Nestor, P. G., 274
Neuman, Alan, 90
neurotransmitters, 46, 102-3, 154, 156, 266-67, 275, 279

NIMH (National Institute of Mental Health), 14, 50-51, 193
nitrogen, 135
nonattachment, 108
nonforgiveness, 183, 215
Non-Kraepelinian Schizophrenia, 276
nonpsychotic major depression, 26, 127, 133-34, 150, 263, 266, 274
NSA (National Security Agency), 78-79

O

'1': The Foundation and Mathematization of Physics (Bedrij), 80
oral triad, 139
oxygen supply, 98, 256
  lack of, 98
Ozawkie Book of the Dead, The (Green), 223

P

paranoia, 17, 132
paranoid schizophrenia, 121, 132, 273
parents, 20, 51, 154-55, 216, 259
  blaming, 170
  children's separation from, 155
  death of, 114
paternal loss, 109
Paul (Christian apostle), 125
peace, 188-89, 195, 197, 200-201, 205-6, 213-14
Pearce, J. C., 266
Peresson violin, 85. *See also* Gabrielli violin
Perior, Patti Damus, 82
Perior, Tim, 82

Philadelphia Psychiatric Center, 88
placebo, 80, 193
plants, 260
powerful voice, 63, 166
preschool children, 33
prevention, three levels of
  prevention of an initial psychosis, 146
  prevention of a recurrence, xiv
  prevention of original trauma, 143
programmed dream
  about loss of a loved one, 239
  complex medical problems solved in, 228
  emergency, 242
  following medical advice received during, 236
  moral issues, 237
  spiritual growth, 243
  techniques, 245
  that ended the Vietnam War, 238
Psychiatric Times, 90
Psychoanalytic Study of the Child, 131
psychosis, 26, 45, 133, 150, 155-56, 161
  acute, 163, 172, 176, 275
  origin of, 225
  preventing the onset of, 52, 100
  regression into, 170
  schizoaffective, 165
  treating, 217
psychotherapy, 173, 175-76, 180, 214
psychotic depression, 17, 53, 127, 133
PTSD (posttraumatic stress disorder), 4-10, 15, 19-21, 23-26, 39, 44-47, 49, 52, 63, 96, 108-9, 112-13, 116, 119, 268-69
  acute, 4-5, 119
  delayed
    from adult life, 23-24, 26

beginning of, 8
from combat, 19, 45
from infancy, xv, 20, 46, 263
onset of, 26
pattern of, 116
positive symptoms of, 39
schizophrenia and, 10, 44
schizophrenia and, 15, 23, 44
survival mechanism in, 20, 45, 116
two types of, 4

Q

Quinn, B., 277

R

rajas, 219
Rama, Swami, 201, 232
Rapp, Doris, 135
Raynaud's phenomenon, 231-32
reality, 51, 179-80, 265
  age of origin of, 98
  age-specific, 100
  See also unreality
regression, 120
  subtle signs of, 169-70
relaxation, 186, 191, 199-200, 202, 204
religion, 76, 80
repression, 8, 21, 24, 26, 31, 34
Risperdal, 159
Ritalin, 134-35
rooting reflex, 101

S

sattva, 219
schizoaffective, 17, 127, 133, 165, 273

schizophrenia
  body movements in, 97
  catatonic, 102, 112, 123, 181
  cause of
    biological change, 115
    facilitating factors, 115
    genetic factors, 106
    migration, 113, 123
    obstetric and birth traumas, 112
    other siblings, 111
    perpetuating factors, 115
    second trimester factors, 109
    stress factors, 112
    time of year born, 110
  childhood, vii, 15, 72, 119, 269
  confirmation of age-of-origin of, 53
  discovery of, 15
  disorganized, 128, 273-74
  hebephrenic, 128
  identical twins with, 107-8
  identifying the age of origin of, 16
  Kraepelinian, 276
  monoamine metabolism in, 277
  negative symptoms in, 23, 53, 273, 277
  non-Kraepelinian, 276
  one common denominator, 18
  paranoid, 121, 132, 273
  positive symptoms in, 23, 53, 277
  precursors of, 23, 25, 41, 43, 146
  purpose of, 20
  simple, 132
  time of year born and, 110, 123
  trap of, 156, 163, 181
"Schizophrenia and the McKenzie Method," 13
Schizophrenia Bulletin, 50
Schlessinger, Laura, 146
school violence, 3, 116, 129-30

Schopenhauer, Arthur, 44
Schweitzer, Albert, 58
science, xviii, 12, 118, 204, 208, 255
Second Annual Report of the King County, 176
second trauma, 45, 52, 114-15, 143, 279
second trimester, 47, 109-10, 123, 255
Selye, Hans, 221
separation trauma, 113, 131, 270
   in drug and alcohol addiction, 138
   flashbacks and, 263
   in infancy, 46, 52, 103, 109, 132
   literature support for, 268
   in preschool children, 33
   schizophrenia and, 48, 53, 118, 132
   in the two-trauma mechanism, 19
serotonin, 17, 183, 194
Shihabuddin, L. S., 276
shock treatment, 98, 179-80, 188-89
Silva, Isabel, 70-71
Silva, Jose, 70, 202
Simonton, Carl, 202
Sivananda Ashram, 81
sleep, xvii, 176, 186
   dreams during, 60-62, 190, 246
   in the laws of the Halacha, 227
   levels of consciousness in, 60
   medical advice during, 236
   meditation and, 202
   in the oral triad, 139
   problem solving in, 250-51
   receiving information during, 219, 224-26, 235, 248
   seeking information during, 61, 76, 222, 227, 248
   visitors appearing in, 244
   words spoken in, 192

Spitz, Rene, 20, 131
Spock, Benjamin, 100
Stachybotrys, 236
starvation, 109, 123, 174, 255
statistical significance, xv, 49, 53, 104-5, 117, 126, 271. *See also* clinical significance
Stevens, Martha Moore, 86
stranger anxiety, 121, 128
stress, 49, 112-13, 120, 136, 196, 205, 221
   factors, 37, 47, 115, 117, 135
   regression as a result of, 101
sucking reflex, 101
suicide, 133-34, 146, 199, 240
survival mechanism, 5, 21, 38, 265
   in PTSD, 7, 45-46, 52, 96
   in schizophrenia, 20
   See also automatic pilot
symbiosis, 119
symbol of infinite oneness, 75, 299. *See also* Trinity ring
symptom expression, 120-21, 128

T

tamas, 219
Taylor, LaDonna, 85-86
telepathy, 89, 258, 260
theory, xiv
   of everything, 80
Therapeutic Alliance, 180-81
theta training, 223
Thorazine, 163
threat, 21, 169, 179
toilet training, 133
total abstinence, 151
transference
   of love energy, 257

thought, 166, 257
transverse myelitis, 231
"trap group," 181
trauma desensitization, 191, 240
traumatic origin, research evidence of, 103
treatment principles, 138, 148, 150-52, 173
Trinity ring, 199, 225, 299. *See also* symbol of infinite oneness
trust, 91, 180
truth, 44, 78, 109, 151, 192, 205
  according to Mahatma Ghandi, 108
  searching for, 58, 76, 118
Turkish Psychological Association, 145
two-trauma mechanism, 18-19, 24, 49, 113-14

U

Ukrainian National Academy of Science, 161
Unintentional Abuse, 127

V

van der Kolk, Bessel A., 269
Ventura, D., 274
viral infections, 110, 123, 278

W

"wall" of the abscess, 8, 25, 39, 41, 53
  penetration of, 36-39, 43, 45
  repression and, 31
  thickening of, 24, 26, 35, 191
Washington DC sniper, 131
Westergaard, T., 111-12
work, 175, 181, 186-87
Wright, Lance, 12, 95, 103, 110
  Delayed Posttraumatic Stress Disorders from Infancy: The Two Trauma Mechanism, xv, 12, 20, 162

The Trinity Ring
A Symbol of Infinite Oneness

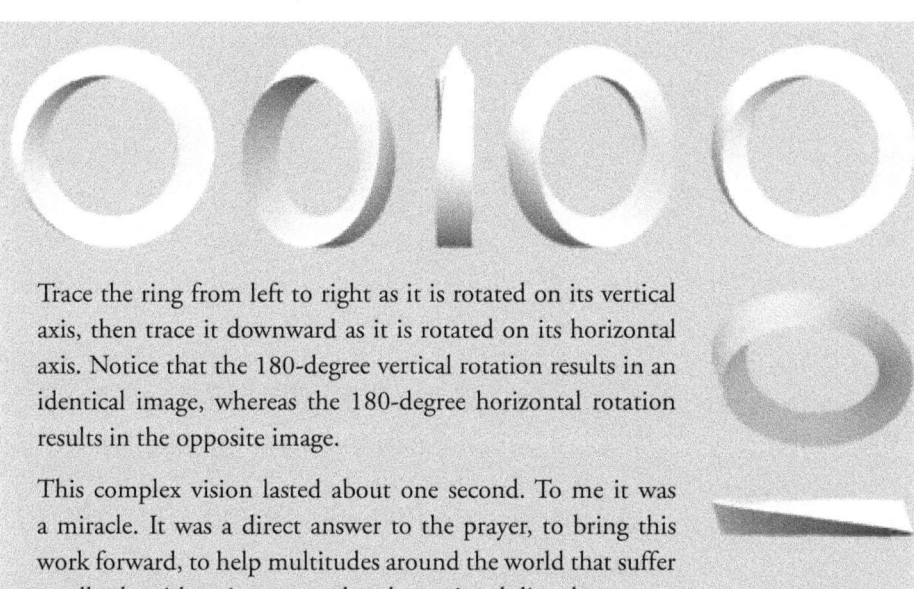

Trace the ring from left to right as it is rotated on its vertical axis, then trace it downward as it is rotated on its horizontal axis. Notice that the 180-degree vertical rotation results in an identical image, whereas the 180-degree horizontal rotation results in the opposite image.

This complex vision lasted about one second. To me it was a miracle. It was a direct answer to the prayer, to bring this work forward, to help multitudes around the world that suffer needlessly with serious mental and emotional disorders.

Many will understand this as a holy symbol, give by God, a Symbol of Infinite Oneness, reminding us that we are one. "May they all be one, as you are in me and I am in you, may they be one in us."

Utility patent number	7,322,211
Design patent numbers:	D551,587
	D560,537
	D559,144

Patented in the United States and the European Nations

www.DrMcKenzie.com

Lightning Source UK Ltd.
Milton Keynes UK
UKHW010022180120
357165UK00001B/36